Stress, Trauma, and Substance Use

T0252825

The editors of *Stress, Trauma, and Substance Use* have gathered a collection of innovative chapters written by cutting edge researchers that depict both the breadth of the relationships between stress, trauma, and substance use, as well as how closely these phenomena are all too often linked.

Individually, the chapters in this volume present innovative conceptual models, original research findings, and recommendations to service providers that are applicable to a diverse body of individuals affected by a wide variety of stressful and/or traumatic experiences, such as HIV/AIDS, incarceration, homelessness, sexual assault, and other forms of trauma and violence in addition to substance use. Taken as a whole, the content of this text provides a window into the true nature of the multi-layered and interconnected relationship between stress, trauma, and substance use. The untangling of these relationships holds great promise for continued research that develops a better understanding of these phenomena and ultimately improves the lives of individuals touched by these experiences.

This book was previously published as a special issue of *Stress, Trauma, and Crisis: An International Journal.*

Brian E. Bride, Ph.D., L.C.S.W. is an Associate Professor of Social Work at the University of Georgia where he conducts research and teaches classes related to clinical practice with substance abuse and mental health, with a particular focus on secondary traumatic stress. His many publications include *Death and Trauma: The Traumatology of Grieving.*

Samuel A. MacMaster, Ph.D. is an Associate Professor of Social Work at the University of Tennessee; the primary focus of his teaching and research has been the intersection of substance use and HIV/AIDS. He has focused specifically on the development of culturally appropriate interventions developed to overcome barriers to service access for underserved populations.

Stress, Trauma, and Substance Use

Edited by Brian E. Bride and
Samuel A. MacMaster

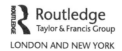

Routledge
Taylor & Francis Group

LONDON AND NEW YORK

First published 2008
by Routledge
2 Park Square, Milton Park, Abingdon, Oxon, OX14 4RN

Simultaneously published in the USA and Canada
by Routledge
270 Madison Avenue, New York, NY 10016

Routledge is an imprint of the Taylor and Francis Group, an informa business

Transferred to Digital Printing 2009

© 2008 Taylor & Francis

Typeset by RefineCatch Limited, Bungay, Suffolk

British Library Cataloguing in Publication Data
A catalogue record for this book is available from the British Library

ISBN10: 0–415–40045–7 (hbk)
ISBN10: 0–415–49560–1 (pbk)

ISBN13: 978–0–415–40045–9 (hbk)
ISBN13: 978–0–415–49560–8 (pbk)

Publisher's Note
The publisher has gone to great lengths to ensure the quality of this reprint
but points out that some imperfections in the original may be apparent.

Contents

Stress, Trauma, and Substance Use: An Overview

BRIAN E. BRIDE

University of Georgia, Athens, Georgia, USA

SAMUEL A. MacMASTER

University of Tennessee, Knoxville, Tennessee, USA

This special issue of *Stress, Trauma, and Crisis: An International Journal* focuses on the interaction between stress, trauma, and substance use. In soliciting manuscripts for this special issue, we cast a deliberately wide net. It would have been relatively easy to compile eight manuscripts that addressed the topic through a myopic lens, such as by focusing only on the assessment and treatment of comorbid posttraumatic stress disorder and substance use disorders. We also could have dictated the type of interaction between the three concepts that we were interested in. For example, we could have specified that manuscripts should address the role of trauma as a risk factor for substance use disorders or the corollary, substance use as a risk factor for traumatic experiences and/or the development of PTSD. Instead, we left it up to the authors to determine how to address the issue of the interaction between stress, trauma, and substance use and where to place the emphasis. Our intention was to provide a forum for innovative manuscripts whose contribution to the literature is found in their unique approach to this interaction and application of empirical investigation to unique problems and/or populations.

Matto presents a review of neuroscientific research on stress vulnerability and its effects on information processing in the context of chemical dependency. This review of basic science explicates the scientific and theoretical underpinnings of an innovative approach to the treatment of chronic chemical dependency. This new approach, the integrated sensory-linguistic model, combines visual processing activities with traditional cognitive-behavioral strategies. The broad goal of this treatment approach is to improve craving management and self-regulation capacities by controlling affective disturbance that arises during visual processing.

Washington and Teague address the issue of suicide among male African-American youth. In particular, they review the literature related to the role of substance use as a risk factor for suicide among this population. In addition, spirituality is discussed as a protective factor that contributes to resiliency in African-American youth. Further, the results of a study that explores the relationship between spirituality and drug attitudes among pre-adolescent African-American males is presented, suggesting the potential for reducing unhealthy drug attitudes through the promotion of spirituality.

According to Holleran and Jung, violence in the form of internalized colonialism, external oppression, and violent acts can be a primary risk factor for negative outcomes such as substance abuse among Mexican-American youth. Many of these youth also must contend with cultural tensions that arise from the acculturative process, role conflicts, school challenges, and identity formation process. However, many Mexican-American adolescents are able to navigate these stressors and traumas in a way that transforms the potentially distressing events into life-affirming rites of passage. Holleran and Jung discuss the results of a qualitative study of Mexican-American youth in a city in the southwestern United States that reveal how these youth utilize their energy, creativity, and resilience to transcend such stressors.

As a life-threatening illness, the diagnosis of HIV or AIDS may be experienced as a traumatic event, while living with HIV/AIDS is experienced by some as a chronic state of stress. Further, certain traumatic experiences are associated with increased risk-behaviors for both HIV/AIDS and substance abuse, and substance use has been found to be a risk factor for certain traumatic experiences and acquiring HIV/AIDS. Jones discusses the complex interaction between chronic stress, traumatic experiences, and substance use among African American women living with HIV/AIDS, the fastest growing demographic of new HIV/AIDS cases. In addition, she presents the results of a qualitative study of African-American women with HIV/AIDS, providing insight into the interaction of the stress of a chronic illness, trauma, and substance use.

Runaway/homeless youth often suffer from exposure to chronic family distress and confront numerous traumatic events in their lives. Further, they face destructive forces that impede their growth such as delinquency, risky sexual experiences, victimization, and violence. Thompson conducted a survey of runaway/homeless youth in New York and Texas to investigate levels of PTSD and the impact of substance use, family, and youth factors on symptom levels. Her results demonstrate heightened rates of trauma symptoms that are predicted by symptoms of depression, anxiety, and dissociation, as well as parental substance use. Based on these results, Thompson argues that runaway/homeless youth entering emergency shelters be evaluated for trauma and associated comorbid symptoms in a manner that recognizes developmental and contextual issues.

Incarcerated women experience high rates of substance abuse disorder and high rates of physical and sexual abuse (Jordan, Schlenger, Fairbank, & Caddell, 1996; Morash, Bynum, & Koons, 1998; Teplin, Abram, & McClelland, 1996). Kubiak, Hanna, and Balton discuss the role of trauma and substance involvement in the lives of incarcerated women by exploring the institutional environment that substance-involved women may encounter during incarceration. In particular, Kubiak and colleagues use a narrative case study approach to describe the stories of three women who experienced sexual assault and/or harassment during their incarceration with a focus on the ways in which they coped with the abuse.

Although the link between trauma and substance use disorders is well documented, assessment and treatment of trauma within substance abuse treatment programs is not often standard practice. Wiechelt and colleagues underline the importance of assessment of traumatic experiences among clients in treatment for substance abuse and report on a two phase project to identify and pilot trauma screening instruments for use in substance abuse treatment settings. The two-phase project was successful in identifying two trauma screening instruments that substance abuse treatment clinicians found to be useful in clinical settings. An additional benefit of Wiechelt and colleagues' efforts is the demonstration of an effective and innovative research-practice collaborative effort.

Comorbidity of PTSD and alcohol use disorders, depression, and physical health problems are well documented (Breslau, Davis, Peterson, & Schultz, 2000; Brown & Wolfe, 1994; Resnick, Acierno, & Kilpatrick, 1997). However, little is known about the occurrence of these problems in persons experiencing trauma symptoms that do not meet the full diagnostic criteria for PTSD. Yarvis and colleagues report on a study that examines the relationship between subthreshold PTSD and alcohol use disorders, depression, and physical health problems in Canadian peacekeepers. Their findings highlight the importance of attending to persons who have experienced traumatic events, but may not meet the full criteria for a diagnosis of PTSD.

This special issue is an addition to the literature that depicts both the breadth of the relationship between stress, trauma, and substance use, as well as how closely these phenomena are linked. These eight articles provide innovative conceptual models, research findings, and recommendations to the practice field that are applied to a diverse body of individuals affected by substance abuse. As individual works they are important, when taken together under this rubric, the true nature of the multi-layered and interconnected relationship between stress and trauma, and substance abuse begins to emerge. It is the untangling of this relationship that the editors of this special issue believe holds great promise for continued research that develops a better understanding of these phenomena and ultimately improves the lives of individuals touched by trauma, crisis, and substance use.

REFERENCES

Breslau, N., Davis, G. C., Peterson, E. L., and Schultz, L. R. (2000). A second look at comorbidity in victims of trauma: The posttraumatic stress disorder—major depression connection. *Biological Psychiatry, 48*, 902–909.

Brown, P. J. and Wolfe, J. (1994). Substance abuse and post-traumatic stress disorder co-morbidity. *Drug and Alcohol Dependency, 35*, 51–59.

Jordan, B. K., Schlenger, W. E., Fairbank, J. A., and Caddell, J. M. (1996). Prevalence of psychiatric disorders among incarcerated women. *Archives of General Psychiatry, 53*, 513–519.

Morash, M., Bynum, T. S., and Koons, B. A. (1998). *Women offenders: Programming needs and promising approaches*. Washington, DC: U.S. Department of Justice, National Institute of Justice.

Resnick, H. S., Acierno, R., and Kilpatrick, D. G. (1997). Health impact of internal personal violence 2: Medical and mental health outcomes. *Behavioral Medicine, 23*, 65–78.

Teplin, L. A., Abram, K. M., and McClelland, G. M. (1996). The prevalence of psychiatric disorder among incarcerated women I: Pre-trial jail detainees. *Archives of General Psychiatry, 53*, 505–512.

1

An Integrated Sensory-linguistic Approach for Drug Addiction: A Synthesis of the Literature and New Directions for Treatment Research

HOLLY C. MATTO

University at Albany, State University of New York, USA

INTRODUCTION

This article synthesizes contemporary neuroscience research on stress vulnerability and its effects on information processing, and is presented as the scientific basis for a new approach to drug-addiction treatment for chronic substance-dependent persons. Research shows that deficits in representational integration, resulting from differences in the way information is processed under extreme stress conditions, requires multi-modal treatment strategies that can accommodate the special learning needs of clients with chronic substance dependency. One new treatment approach, an integrated sensory-linguistic model based on dual representation theory, is introduced. This treatment model encourages clients to take hold of the sensory and emotional elements related to the addiction process through in vivo visual processing experiences that are integrated with cognitive-behavioral techniques, rather than leaving this material vulnerable to implicit activation by environmental triggers. The treatment model's direct linkage to this contemporary body of scientific research is explicated. The paper concludes by outlining important new opportunities for research on stress vulnerability and addiction.

LITERATURE REVIEW

Animal studies have shown that drug-seeking behavior is precipitated by five factors: 1) conditioned stimuli; 2) stress; 3) withdrawal; 4) drug injection; and 5) electrical brain stimulation (Spanagel, 2003, p. 297). Presented is a review of the literature on the factors specific to a stress vulnerability model of chronic drug addiction—conditioned stimuli, neural stress trajectory, and withdrawal.

Conditioned Stimuli

Research studies examining conditioned stimuli and cue reactivity have shown that desire to drink severity and physiological reactivity are strongly associated with relapse rate (Cooney, Litt, Morse, Bauer, & Gaupp, 1997); and drug cravings have been found to be strongly associated with drug cue reactivity from conditioned stimuli (Glautier & Drummond, 1994), suggesting the need for treatment approaches to focus on coping with cravings and managing cue reactivity in order to decrease the risk of relapse. Negative mood states have been found to significantly increase craving for drugs/alcohol (Litt, Cooney, Kadden, & Gaupp, 1990; Quigley & Marlatt, 1999; Robbins, Ehrman, Childress, Cornish, & O'Brien, 2000), which, in turn, increase relapse potential. Along these lines, Cooney et al. (1997) state a need for developing "treatment methods that help [cue] reactors reduce their responsiveness to negative mood states and to stimuli in the environment" (p. 249), indicating the importance of attending to both internal (physiological and psychological) and external (context-dependent) cues for treatment focus. Thus, attention to the specific internal as well as environmental cues that leave an addicted person with marked vulnerability to relapse is a salient component of any treatment program for addicted persons struggling in the early stages of recovery.

Neural Stress Trajectory and Withdrawal

Neuroscientists specializing in drug addiction have found that cravings result from an increasingly hyperaroused neural system that, with progressed substance use, enhances the urge to use and produces strong motivation to initiate drug-seeking behavior (Koob & Le Moal, 1996; Robinson & Berridge, 1993). "A second and potentially independent pathway may induce alcohol craving and relapse by negative motivational states, including conditioned withdrawal and stress. This pathway seems to involve the glutamatergic system and the corticotropin-releasing hormone (CRH)-system. Chronic alcohol intake leads to compensatory changes within these systems. During withdrawal and abstinence, increased glutamatergic excitatory neurotransmission as well as increased CRH release lead to a state of hyperexcitability that becomes manifest as craving, anxiety, seizures, and autonomic dysregulation" (Spanagel, 2003, p. 298).

This stress trajectory initially develops in the hypothalamic-pituitary-adrenal (HPA) axis which, when activated, releases corticotropin-releasing hormone (CRH) and, ultimately, glucocorticoid hormones (cortisol), leading to heightened vulnerability to drug-seeking behaviors. Recent animal studies have found that drug-seeking behavior can be reduced by blocking CRH levels using a CRH antagonist and by controlling the stress hormone corticosterone (cortisol in humans; Marinelli & Piazza, 2003), demonstrating that "CRHR1 activation contributes to foot-shock stress-induced reinstatement of alcohol seeking via its action on extrahypothalamic sites" (Spanagel, 2003, p. 305).

Other studies that have examined disruption in this fear-stress system suggest that when glutamate levels are significantly increased in the amygdala, resulting from engagement with drug-related stimuli, the neural circuitry becomes hyperaroused (Quertemont, de Neuville, & De Witte, 1998), indicating that substance-related conditioned stimuli create a biological stress reaction that can motivate behavior to alleviate the negative state. Prolonged substance use that produces chronic stress on the biological system, such as repeated drug use—withdrawal cycles that create patterned and persistent system dysregulation, heightens reactivity to conditioned stimuli and increases the risk of relapse. This neurophysiological dysregulation provides a biological understanding for why stress and concomitant problematic affect are two of the most significant predictors of substance abuse relapse (Brewer, Catalano, Haggerty, Gainey, & Fleming, 1998); with some researchers indicating problematic affect/emotions account for 35% of relapse episodes (Quigley & Marlatt, 1999). The next section on information processing further explains the impact of this neural stress trajectory on learning, memory and behavior for persons with chronic drug addiction.

Information Processing

In addition to the direct impact of stress on biological arousal and craving reactivity, research shows stress related to substance use and withdrawal profoundly disrupts the body's natural ability to modulate subsequent stress response (leading to heightened and persistent excitation), and that this directly influences *information* (representations originating from interaction with stimuli; Massaro & Cowan, 1993) *processing* (flow of information through a system; Massaro & Cowan, 1993) which, then, influences learning and memory.

A recent study by Saal, Dong, Bonci, and Malenk (2003) found exposure to stress itself (without concomitant exposure to drugs) induced long-term potentiation (LTP) (synaptic mechanism responsible for associational learning that strengthens future learned response to an activating stimulus; Teyler & DiScenna, 1987), similar to LTP induction caused by addictive drugs alone (i.e., alcohol, nicotine, cocaine, amphetamine, morphine). These results show that the stress trajectory and its conditioning properties mimicked the drug trajectory and its conditioning properties, and suggests that stress alone may create vulnerability to past addiction reminders and may motivate drug-seeking behaviors. These researchers suggest that a priming effect (where previously-learned material increases the efficiency in responding to similar information in the future) is evidenced; whereby, stress itself mimics the pathway of previous drug-use experiences and, therefore, contributes to heightened drug-seeking motivation.

Schacter, Chiu, and Ochsner (1993) and Squire, Knowlton, and Musen (1993) work indicates that "perceptual priming" works independent of declarative (conscious processing) memory, and that such stimuli can have a long-term effect on behavior. In addition, the distinct perceptual features of the stimuli (e.g., image, sound, tone, etc.) will influence the reinstatement process between the new stimuli and previous stimuli experience. Taken together, these findings indicate that chronic substance dependent persons who experience extreme stress independent of and/or related to their addiction may have addiction reminders (e.g., conditioned stimuli) stored as learned responses that are not consciously processed (i.e., non-declarative memories) that become vulnerable to activation at this implicit or non-declarative level.

Further, strong emotional arousal that occurs during stress-induced experiences has been shown to strengthen the implicated neural circuitry and, therefore, enhance memory encoding of the stress experience, creating a strong learned response—a phenomenon Daniel Schacter (2001) calls "persistence." As such, emotionally intense substance-related experiences (associated with withdrawal, risky drug-seeking behaviors, etc.) are likely to strengthen biologically wired non-declarative memories of these experiences. The brain's natural response to this neural excitation that occurs at the time of a significant stress experience is the release of gamma-aminobutyric acid (GABA), a synaptic inhibitor that dampens the excitatory response in the amygdala. However, conditioned stimuli associated with strong emotional arousal derived from previous learning associations and developed over time (conditioned responses that become automatic) can negate GABAs inhibitory effects and maintain anxiety. Specifically, the stress hormone cortisol has been found to limit GABA's ability to inhibit glutamate's excitatory response (LeDoux, 2002; Spanagel, 2003), suggesting that increased stress, which increases the release of cortisol and weakens the inhibiting effect of GABA on glutamate, may exacerbate a state of heightened excitation. This has been shown in drug addiction studies where the neural excitation that occurs during withdrawal has been associated with impaired GABA transmission (Morrow, Montpied, Lingford-Hughes, Paul, 1990; Petrie et al., 2001).

Of particular interest in understanding disruption in information processing and, thus, learning and memory processes associated with drug addiction, are the two central functions of the hippocampus: 1) its contextualizing function; and 2) its capacity for forming explicit or declarative (consciously accessible) memories. Research shows the hippocampus plays a critical role in providing the amygdala (site where fear conditioning occurs and the structure that evaluates stimuli) with information about the context where emotional learning transpires (LeDoux, 2002; Siegel, 1999), projecting the information to the prefrontal region (where reasoning, abstraction and higher levels of cognitive functioning take place), allowing for increased cortical control over amygdalar excitation and the fear response.

The prefrontal region, specifically, functions to coordinate information across sensory modalities, memory, and emotional circuitry in order to translate the experience into temporal and contextual awareness and, therefore, regulates the significance of the stress experience. However, if there is a disconnect in circuitry between and among these structures—the prefrontal region, hippocampus, and amygdala—as studies have found to occur during intense emotional arousal that impairs hippocampal functioning and shuts the frontal lobe off-line, then implicit or non-declarative (out of conscious awareness) storage of arousal experiences may occur.

Therefore, with hippocampal impairment, forming explicit or declarative (consciously accessible) memories will be inhibited (Squire, 1987, 1992; Squire & Zola-Morgan, 1991; Zola-Morgan & Squire, 1993). Studies show that extreme stress experiences disrupt explicit memory processing as an increase in cortisol decreases the glucose in hippocampal neurons resulting in heightened sensitivity to the excitatory properties of glutamate. Hippocampal cells in the CA3 region may, then, shrink and die off in reaction to low glucose (energy) levels, causing overall hippocampal volume shrinkage, impaired capacity to form explicit memory, and an inability to properly contextualize sensory-based stimuli, leading to implicit (conditioned automatic learned responses) processing of external experience that affect self-regulation capacities (LeDoux, 2002).

Hippocampal impairment, as has been found after repeated alcohol withdrawals (Veatch & Gonzales, 1996), and the subsequent implicit processing of extreme stress experiences, coupled with Spanagel (2003) research that shows increased "glutamatergic excitatory neurotransmission" can lead to drug cravings, indicates that sensory-based cue triggers may remain out of "explicit" conscious awareness, and reinforces the importance of multi-modal processing approaches, suggesting that CBT is a necessary but perhaps not sufficient treatment method for chronic substance-dependent persons.

More specifically, Morris, Ohman, and Dolan (1998) found that the visual-processing centers in the brain were uniquely affected by amygdala excitation during stress conditioning, showing that visual sensory stimuli were more likely to be stored implicitly, rather than explicitly, during the conditioning process when the amygdala is intensely emotionally aroused. This suggests that multi-modal treatment approaches that focus on access to sensory-based, implicitly-stored experiences should include a substantial visual-processing component. Because hippocampal structural changes may be slow to evolve over time, resulting from periods of repeated and chronic exposure to extreme stress conditions, chronic "hard-to-treat" substance-dependent persons who experience such extreme stress over long periods of time may be particularly vulnerable to such structural and functional changes. As such, this target group is hypothesized to significantly benefit from a new multimodal treatment approach that responds to this neurophysiological vulnerability and matches this information-processing trajectory.

DUAL REPRESENTATION THEORY

In guiding new multimodal treatment developments for substance abuse, one information-processing theory, dual representation theory, is particularly useful. Dual representation theory has developed from this science base and has been used to understand extreme stress disorders such as posttraumatic stress disorder (PTSD; Brewin, 2001; Brewin, Dalgleish, & Joseph, 1996). Based on the research that shows that representations of experiences under high stress conditions become processed implicitly in the body, as opposed to being linguistically processed, dual representation theory posits two memory systems that need to be addressed in treatment: 1) verbally accessible memories (VAM), which are consciously retrieved and temporally contextualized; and 2) situationally accessible memory (SAM), which are signified by perceptual information (e.g, images, sensations, etc.) that lack conscious retrieval capacity (Brewin, 2001). SAM, or what other researchers have called "implicit" memory (Siegel, 1999; Siegel, 2003; Solomon & Siegel, 2003; Squire, 1987, 1992; van der Kolk, McFarlane, & Weisaeth, 1996), "nondeclarative" memory (Milner, Squire, & Kandel, 1998; Squire et al., 1993; van der Kolk et al. 1996) or "somatosensory information" (Eckberg, 2000), are stored in the body as a result of hampered neocortical (frontal lobe) functioning at the time of extreme stress (Rothchild, 2000; Schore, 1994) and include conditioned learned responses.

Persistent extreme stress cycles, as is the case with chronic drug dependency, continue to keep experiences represented in the body as sensory states, without concomitant cognitive representation, leaving them vulnerable to activation and retrieval by exposure to similar sensory cues. For example, drug dreams that are common with chronic substance-dependent persons in early recovery is an example of how intrusive memory of past drug-related experiences can deeply affect the human system on multiple sensory levels that may operate out of consciousness. To this end, dual-representation theory and current neuroscience research on substance abuse suggest that treatment approaches that incorporate sensory-based techniques, such as directed visual-processing techniques, that are integrated with traditional cognitive-based techniques are important developments to pursue. By reinstating previously impaired cortical processes with the triggered sensory state through the application of CBT strategies during the sensory-based expressive process, the individual may gain access to a wider repertoire of emotional and behavioral response options.

Thus, the broad treatment goal is to facilitate activation of these implicit experiences to gain greater cognitive control over them, rather than allowing them to remain as automatic responses left out of conscious awareness and susceptible to activation in the future by similar sensory-based triggers. In facilitating the development of cortical plasticity necessary to engage declarative memory capacities, modification of these representations becomes possible. Accessing the implicitly encoded experiences through sensory-based methods and then transforming those experiences through activation of the prefrontal region (using CBT techniques) can facilitate the integration necessary for achieving self-regulation.

INTEGRATED SENSORY-LINGUISTIC MODEL

This impressive body of research provides compelling evidence that new multi-modal treatment methods are needed to meet the unique learning needs of clients who have experienced extreme stress conditions such as severe trauma (e.g., PTSD) and chronic substance dependence. This integrated sensory-linguistic treatment approach combines visual processing activities with traditional CBT strategies, such as self-monitoring, cognitive restructuring, and behavioral rehearsal, to help individuals recognize and manage drug cravings through a multi-modal processing system that includes access to somatosensory conditioned cues. The broad goal of treatment is to improve craving management and self-regulation capacities by controlling affective disturbances that arise during visual processing. This is done by expanding the client's capacity to access and express multimodal representations of experience through the visual activity, and by strengthening new associative cortical connections during CBT processing.

Engaging the client in sensory cue exploration (addiction reminders) can serve to recontextualize the information in a recovery environment, developing new recovery-related associations that contradict the past associative context (highly arousing and fear-based), and increase cognitive flexibility and control. Integrating visual-processing techniques into traditional

CBT protocols allows emotional, bodily, and visual representations of experience to become accessible in a controlled environment. The introduction of cognitive-regulation strategies to contain the accessed sensory-based cues provides an opportunity to alter their intensity and reactive power. Research shows that if these conditioned responses that have been stored as sensory-based material in the body are not accessed, the system remains vulnerable to response activation in the future by stimuli that matches the encoded material (e.g., sights, smells, sensations that mimic the drug-related stored experiences; Brewin, 2001; Brewin et al., 1996; Cozolino, 2002; Eckberg, 2000; Rothchild, 2000; Siegel, 1999; van der Kolk et al., 1996).

Changes in the individual's reactivity capacity are sought by modifying response activation through enhancing cortical control over the sensory stimuli through increased focal attention during visual expression, leading to decreased vulnerability to these triggers and to improved mood stability. Dual-representation theory suggests that without initial access to this sensory material, CBT and cortical processing alone may be less effective in this early treatment stage. "Learning to use neocortical reasoning abilities to observe and then intervene in reflexive initial dyregulatory responses is often a helpful approach... the neocortex can override these responses and bring the deeper structures into a more tolerable level of arousal. This can be accomplished by any number of 'self-talk' strategies in which imagery, internal dialogue and evocative memory can be activated" (Siegel, 1999, p. 275).

This approach is consistent with current research that emphasizes the importance of bilateral integration across brain hemispheres for consolidation of information that has initially failed to respond to cortical processing and storage (e.g., external and internal drug cues that are stored in the body and can be easily triggered by sensory cues), and for strengthening self-organizing capacities (Cozolino, 2002; Siegel, 1999). Visually expressive experiences can help facilitate self-organization by activating mental imagery that is experienced through the different sensory modalities in the body and expressed through the creative process (Malchiodi, 2003). The intense emotional arousal, as that which can arise during implementation of sensory-based expressive techniques, activates multiple brain regions increasing the opportunity in treatment for coordinated and integrated learning to take place. Specifically, techniques such as "journal writing, guided imagery, and exercises for 'drawing on the right side of the brain' have proven helpful to catelyze such a new form of bilateral resonance" (Siegel, 1999, p. 237).

CURRENT RESEARCH ON INTEGRATIVE APPROACHES

As shown, researchers and clinicians assert that mental health comes from integrating differentiated parts of the brain, such as connecting the limbic system with front lobe (emotion and cognition); facilitating "bilateral integration" (left-right hemisphere), and temporal integration (past, present and future representations; Siegel, 1999; Solomon & Siegel, 2003; van der Kolk, 2002). The next section will review the current treatment research that uses integrated psychosocial approaches to work towards these goals.

Pollack et al.'s (2002) recent treatment-effectiveness study findings offer support for the importance of attending to "interoceptive" or affect-laden cues associated with substance use in order to decrease the likelihood of using illicit drugs post-treatment. Specifically, Pollack et al. (2002) employed a new CBT treatment protocol that included a component targeting interoceptive cues, originally employed to treat patients with panic disorder, with an opiate-dependent sample of patients receiving methadone ($N = 23$). These researchers found that cognitive-restructuring strategies combined with interoceptive cue exposure was found to be more effective than standard care alone in reducing substance use, but was more effective for women in their sample as compared to men (Pollack et al., 2002). Similarly, other researchers have found that visual and olfactory cue exposure techniques are effective in delaying relapse for alcohol-dependent persons, but do not make gender-specific claims (Drummond & Glautier, 1994; Glautier & Drummond, 1994).

Other novel treatment approaches that integrate CBT techniques with multi-modal interventions have recently been developed to target cues and manage symptomology in special substance abuse populations. Back, Dansky, Carroll, Foa, and Brady (2001) developed a manualized treatment approach that integrated imaginal and in-vivo exposure therapy with cognitive-behavioral techniques for persons with co-occurring PTSD and cocaine-dependency. The researchers' preliminary study found that both PTSD symptoms and cocaine use were reduced at post-treatment, for those patients who completed the integrated treatment protocol, and that these patients were able to sustain the gains when assessed at six-month follow-up (Brady, Dansky, Back, Foa, & Carroll, 2001). This study provides new preliminary evidence that exposure therapy for some substance abuse populations does not increase the risk for relapse, as previous admonitions against exposure therapy had suggested.

These promising results are consistent with other studies that have shown in-treatment stress activation, as demonstrated via exposure techniques, is necessary to access the implicated neural networks associated with the conditioned fear response (Blakely & Baker, 1980; Hodgson & Rankin, 1983; Jacobs & Nadel, 1985; McLellan, Childress, Ehrman, & O'Brien, 1986). Moderate levels of stress are important in facilitating neural changes that strengthen learning and cortical restructuring (Cowan & Kandel, 2001; Zhu & Waite, 1998). Stress, when activated in a structured therapeutic setting, may provide the biological state conducive to neural network reorganization and, as such, may be a necessary condition for biobehavioral change. Results across these various studies indicate that continued examination of a variety of exposure and expressive therapeutic techniques as integrated with traditional CBT, such as those described in this sensory-linguistic treatment approach, is important for expanding behavioral treatment developments with various substance abuse populations.

Integrating CBT techniques with structured visually expressive activities have been successfully employed with other mental health conditions. William Steele and colleagues tested the effectiveness of a structured trauma intervention that integrated drawing with CBT techniques, as part of a grant from the National Institute for Trauma and Loss in Children. The intervention, which included exposure to traumatic material facilitated by drawing activities, helped children construct a trauma narrative from the drawing experience and to modify the narrative through cognitive reframing (Steele, 2003; Steele & Raider, 2001). Study results showed the intervention that combined structured drawing techniques with cognitive reframing decreased trauma symptomology in three specific categories: "reexperiencing, avoidance, and arousal" (Steele, 2003, p. 139; Steele & Raider, 2001). Improvements were similar for all levels of trauma severity. This study contributes additional empirical support for the use of structured sensory-based techniques, such as visual directives, in treating conditions that originate from extreme stress experiences, that are characterized by intense system arousal, and that include triggered states. The study demonstrates that drawing activities effectively facilitate exposure to stored material that can be surfaced and modified through subsequent application of cognitive techniques.

NEW EMPIRICAL INQUIRY

Empirical studies designed to test new multi-modal treatments that respond in a new way to this neural stress trajectory and facilitate left-right hemisphere integration, are needed. In addition, such studies should examine how stress severity interacts with treatment effectiveness (e.g., do those patients with higher stress levels benefit more from this treatment approach). Specifically, new research should test whether an integrated sensory-linguistic treatment approach for chronic substance-dependent persons is more effective at improving patient self-regulation capacities by managing cravings and reducing affective disturbances, than cortical processing alone (traditional cognitive-behavioral therapy [CBT] only). Exploratory research questions might include: Do chronic substance-dependent persons who participate in the integrated sensory-linguistic treatment approach demonstrate better self-regulation capacities as compared to persons who participate in the CBT-only standard care treatment? If significant effects are found, are they related to subject attributes of gender or stress severity? If significant effects are found, is there evidence of a dosage effect (i.e., does self-regulation improvement significantly correlate with dosage (LOS: number of sessions; length of sessions) of treatment condition?).

Testing for potential gender differences is important as other similar studies have demonstrated significant differences in effectiveness for women as compared to men (see Pollack et al., 2002), and because research studies have shown differential rates of affective disturbance for drug-dependent men and women (Jung, 2001; Kandel, Warner, & Kessler, 1998). Women with drug dependency have shown higher rates of concomitant anxiety and affective disturbance as compared to drug-dependent men, suggesting that treatment approaches that target affective self-regulation capacities, like this sensory-linguistic treatment approach, may show differential effectiveness across gender. Stress severity is identified as a potentially important subject attribute as it is consistent with the theoretical and scientific basis presented in the literature review, which suggests that chronic substance-dependent persons show a neural stress trajectory that affects self-regulation capacities. Examining potential interaction effects between stress, drug abuse, and multi-modal treatment approaches is an important and intriguing area of further study.

CONCLUSION

If learning alters synaptic connections as the neuroscience research over the decades has shown, then psychosocial treatment, as a learning process, can alter such synaptic connections (Cozolino, 2002; LeDoux, 2002; Siegel, 1999; Solomon & Siegel, 2003). In as much as psychosocial treatments are able to change the synaptic connections in the brain via new learning experiences (Kandel & Squire, 1992) and grow new integrative fibers (Solomon & Siegel, 2003) through new learning experiences, new behavioral response options become available. It is in the fine-tuning of our understanding of how specific treatment components change specific synaptic connections (and effect learning) for specific biopsychosocial conditions that focuses future empirical study. This paper presented the scientific and theoretical underpinnings of a new treatment approach for chronic substance-dependent persons, a sensory-linguistic model, and encourages new treatment research in this area of stress vulnerability and drug addiction.

REFERENCES

Back, S. E., Dansky, B. S., Carroll, K. M., Foa, E. B., and Brady, K. T. (2001). Exposure therapy in the treatment of PTSD among cocaine-dependent individuals: Description of procedures. *Journal of Substance Abuse Treatment, 21*(1), 35–45.

Blakely, R. and Baker, R. (1980). An exposure approach to alcohol abuse. *Behavior Research and Therapy, 84,* 319–325.

Brady, K. T., Dansky, B. S., Back, S. E., Foa, E. B., and Carroll, K. M. (2001). Exposure therapy in the treatment of PTSD among cocaine-dependent individuals: Preliminary findings. *Journal of Substance Abuse Treatment, 21*(1), 47–54.

Brewer, D. D., Catalano, R. F., Haggerty, K., Gainey, R. R., and Fleming, C. B. (1998). A meta-analysis of predictors of continued drug use during and after treatment for opiate addiction. *Addiction, 93*, 73–92.

Brewin, C. R. (2001). A cognitive neuroscience account of posttraumatic stress disorder and its treatment. *Behaviour Research and Therapy, 39*, 373–393.

Brewin, C. R., Dagleish, T., and Joseph, S. (1996). A dual representation theory of posttraumatic stress disorder. *Psychological Review, 103*(4), 670–686.

Cooney, N. L., Litt, M. D., Morse, P. A., Bauer, L. O., and Gaupp, L. (1997). Alcohol cue reactivity, negative-mood reactivity, and relapse in treated alcoholic men. *Journal of Abnormal Psychology, 106*(2), 243–250.

Cowan, W. M. and Kandel, E. R. (2001). A brief history of synapses and synaptic transmission. In W. M. Cowan, T. C. Sudhof, & C. F. Stevens (Eds.), *Synapses* (pp. 1–87). Baltimore: Johns Hopkins University Press.

Cozolino, L. (2000). *The neuroscience of psychotherapy.* New York: Norton.

Drummond, D. C. and Glautier, S. (1994). A controlled trial of cue exposure treatment in alcohol dependence. *Journal of Consulting and Clinical Psychology, 62*, 809–817.

Eckberg, M. (2000). *Victims of cruelty: Somatic psychotherapy in the treatment of Posttraumatic Stress Disorder.* Berkeley, CA: North Atlantic Books.

Glautier, S. and Drummond, D. C. (1994). Alcohol dependence and cue reactivity. *Journal of Studies on Alcohol, 55*, 224–229.

Hodgson, R. J. and Rankin, H. J. (1983). Cue exposure and relapse prevention. In W. M. Hay & P. E. Nathan (Eds.), *Clinical case studies in the behavioral treatment of alcoholism* (pp. 207–226). New York: Plenum.

Jacobs, W. and Nadel, L. (1985). Stress-induced recovery of fears and phobias. *Psychological Review, 92*(4), 512–531.

Jung, J. (2001). *Psychology of alcohol and other drugs.* Thousand Oaks, CA: Sage.

Kandel, E. R. and Squire, L. R. (1992). Cognitive neuroscience. *Current Opinion in Neurobiology, 2*, 143–145.

Kandel, D. B., Warner, L. A., and Kessler, R. C. (1998). The epidemiology of substance use and dependence among women. In C. L. Wetherington & A. B. Roman (Eds.), *Drug addiction research and the health of women* (pp. 105–130). Washington, DC: National Institute on Drug Abuse.

Koob, G. F. and Le Moal, M. (1996). Drug abuse: Hedonic homeostatic dysregulation. *Science, 278*, 52–58.

LeDoux, J. E. (2002). *Synaptic self: How our brains become who we are.* New York: Penguin Books.

Litt, M. D., Cooney, N. L., Kadden, R. M., and Gaupp, L. (1990). Reactivity to alcohol cues and induced moods in alcoholics. *Addictive Behaviors, 15*(2), 137–146.

Malchiodi, C. (2003). Art therapy and the brain. In C. A. Malchiodi (Ed.), *Handbook of art therapy* (pp. 16–24). New York: Guilford.

Marinelli, M. and Piazza, P. V. (2003). Influence of environmental and hormonal factors in sensitivity to psychostimulants. In R. Maldonado (Ed.), *Molecular biology of drug addiction* (pp. 133–159). Totowa, NJ: Humana Press.

Massaro, D. W. and Cowan, N. (1993). Information processing models: Microscopes of the mind. *Annual Review of Psychology, 44*, 383–425.

McLellan, A. T., Childress, A. R., Ehrman, R., and O'Brien, C. P. (1986). Extinguishing conditioned responses during opiate treatment: Turning laboratory findings into clinical procedures. *Journal of Substance Abuse Treatment, 3*, 33–40.

Milner, B., Squire, L. R., and Kandel, E. R. (1998). Cognitive neuroscience and the study of memory. *Neuron, 20*, 445–468.

Morris, J. S., Ohman, A., and Dolan, R. J. (1998). Conscious and unconscious emotional learning in the human amygdala. *Nature, 393*, 467–470.

Morrow, A. L., Montpied, P., Lingford-Hughes, A., and Paul, S. M. (1990). Chronic ethanol and pentobarbital administration in the rat: Effects on GABA receptor function and expression in the brain. *Alcohol, 7*, 237–244.

Petrie, J., Sapp, D. W., Tyndale, R. F., Park, M. K., Fanselow, M., and Olson, R. W. (2001). Altered GABA receptor subunit and splice variant expression in rats treated with chronic intermittent ethanol. *Alcoholism: Clinical and Experimental Research, 25*(6), 819–828.

Pollack, M. H., Penava, S. A., Bolton, E., Worthington, J. J., Allen, G. L., Farach, F. J., and Otto, M. W. (2002). A novel cognitive-behavioral approach for treatment-resistant drug dependence. *Journal of Substance Abuse Treatment, 23*(4), 335–342.

Quertemont, E., de Neuville, J., and De Witte, P. (1998). Changes in the amygdala amino acid microdialysate after conditioning with a cue associated with ethanol. *Psychopharmacology, 139*, 71–78.

Quigley, L. A. and Marlatt, G. A. (1999). Relapse prevention: Maintenance of change after initial treatment. In B. S. McCrady & E. E. Epstein (Eds.), *Addictions: A comprehensive guidebook* (pp. 370–384). New York: Oxford University Press.

Robbins, S. J., Ehrman, R. N., Childress, A. R., Cornish, J. W., and O'Brien, C. P. (2000). Mood state and recent cocaine use are not associated with levels of cocaine cue reactivity. *Drug and Alcohol Dependence, 59*(1), 33–42.

Robinson, T. E. and Berridge, K. C. (1993). The neural base of drug craving: an incentive-sensitization theory of addiction. *Brain Research Reviews, 18*, 247–291.

Rothchild, B. (2000). *The body remembers: The psychophysiology of trauma and trauma treatment*. New York: Norton.

Saal, D., Dong, Y., Bonci, A., and Malenka, R. (2003). Drugs of abuse and stress trigger a common synaptic adaptation in dopamine neurons. *Neuron, 37*(4), 577–582.

Schacter, D. L. (2001). *The seven sins of memory*. Boston: Houghton Mifflin.

Schacter, D. L., Chiu, C.-Y. P., and Ochsner, K. N. (1993). Implicit memory: A selective review. *Annual Review of Neuroscience, 16*, 159–182.

Schore, A. (1994). *Affect regulation and the origin of the self*. Hillsdale, NJ: Erlbaum.

Siegel, D. (1999). *The developing mind*. New York: Guilford.

Siegel, D. (2003). An interpersonal neurobiology of psychotherapy: The developing mind and the resolution of trauma. In M. Solomon & D. Siegel (Eds.), *Healing trauma: Attachment, mind, body, and brain* (pp. 1–56). New York: Norton.

Solomon, M. F. and Siegel, D. J. (2003). *Healing trauma*. New York: W. W. Norton.

Spanagel, R. (2003). Behavioral and molecular aspects of alcohol craving and relapse. In R. Maldonado (Ed.), *Molecular biology of drug addiction* (pp. 295–313). Totowa, NJ: Humana Press.

Squire, L. R. (1987). *Memory and brain*. New York: Oxford University Press.

Squire, L. R. (1992). Declarative and non-declarative memory: Multiple brain systems supporting learning and memory. *Journal of Cognitive Neuroscience, 4,* 232–243.

Squire, L. R., Knowlton, B., and Musen, G. (1993). The structure and organization of memory. *Annual Review of Psychology, 44,* 453–495.

Squire, L. R. and Zola-Morgan, S. (1991). The medial temporal lobe memory system. *Science, 153,* 2380–2386.

Steele, W. (2003). Using drawing in short-term trauma resolution. In C. A. Malchiodi (Ed.), *Handbook of art therapy* (pp. 139–151). New York: Guilford.

Steele, W. and Raider, M. (2001). *Structured sensory interventions for traumatized children, adolescents, and parents: Strategies to alleviate trauma.* New York: Edwin Mellen Press.

Teyler, T. J. and DiScenna, P. (1987). Long-term potentiation. *Annual Review of Neuroscience, 10,* 131–161.

van der Kolk, B. A. (2002). Beyond the talking cure: Somatic experience and subcortical imprints in the treatment of trauma. In F. Shapiro (Ed.), *EMDR as an integrative psychotherapy approach* (pp. 57–83). Washington, DC: American Psychiatric Association.

van der Kolk, B. A., McFarlane, A. C., and Weisaeth, L. (1996). *Traumatic stress.* New York: Guilford.

Veatch, L. M. and Gonzales, L. P. (1996). Repeated ethanol withdrawal produces site-dependent increases in EEG spiking. *Alcoholism: Clinical and Experimental Research, 20,* 262–267.

Zhu, X. O. and Waite, P. M. E. (1998). Cholinergic depletion reduces plasticity of barrel field cortex. *Cerebral Cortex, 8,* 63–72.

Zola-Morgan, S. and Squire, L. (1993). The neuroanatomy of memory. *Annual Review of Neuroscience, 16,* 547–563.

2

Young African-American Male Suicide Prevention and Spirituality

GREGORY WASHINGTON and KATHERYN TEAGUE

University of Tennessee College of Social Work, Memphis, Tennessee, USA

INTRODUCTION

The rates of suicide in the United States among all pre-adolescents and adolescents have doubled over the last few decades. This is particularly true among African-American youth, whose suicide rates have historically been lower than European-American youth. Between 1980 and 1995, a total of 3,030 African Americans aged 10–19 years committed suicide (CDC, 1998). This reflects a 114% increase for African Americans aged 10–19 years, with the largest increase (233%) being among African Americans aged 10–14 years as compared to a 120% increase for their European Americans counter-parts. Among all African Americans aged 15–19 years, the suicide rate increased 126%, compared with 19% for European-American youth. Among African-American males aged 15–19 years, the suicide rate increased 146%, compared with 22% for European-American males of the same age group. The troubling nature of this sudden increase is made more mysterious by recent research findings by Goldsmith, Pellmar, Kleinman, and Bunney (2002) of the Institute of Medicine that indicate recent suicide rates among

African-American males are declining. This could mean concerns about a developing African-American male suicide crisis are unwarranted.

Little is known about the onset and characteristics of suicide risk factors that are particularly relevant to African-American youth. This is further complicated because reporting suicide and suicide attempts is non-uniform across jurisdictions (Goldsmith et al., 2002). There are only a few scholars that have considered whether hypotheses derived from suicide studies of European Americans are applicable to African Americans (Bell & Clark, 1998; Mazza & Reynolds, 1999; Nisbet, 1996). The limited analysis of applicability to African Americans is also true of prevention programs that attempt to address the risk of suicide among African-American youth. Few of these programs address risk factors unique to African-American youth (CDC, 1998; Garland & Zigler, 1993). While there are several potential risk factors for suicide that warrant attention, substance abuse as a risk factor for young African-American male suicide will be the focus of this article.

RISK FACTORS

The epidemiological literature has shown that the young African-American males in poor communities could to be at the greatest risk for suicide (CDC, 1998; Gibbs, 1997; Reid, Lee, Jedlicka, & Shin, 1977). A factor that is associated with an increased risk for suicide includes substance abuse (Rich, Fowler, Fogarty, & Young, 1998). Direct influences related to substance abuse by African-American youth and indirect influences related to substance abuse by family members of African-American youth are purported to increase their risk of suicide.

Although research has shown that African-American youth were less likely or no more likely to be users of illicit drugs than European-American youth (De La Rosa, Segal, & Lopez, 1999; Wallace, Brown, Bachman, & Laveist, 2003), their involvement in drug-related activities is important for at least two reasons. First, drug use typically increases in the middle of adolescence for all youth, particularly males (Chipungu et al., 2000). At the same time, the National Household Survey on Drug Abuse in 2001 indicates a modest increase among youth 12 and 13 (U.S. Department of Health and Human Services, 2002).

Second, African Americans irrespective of age have been found to experience greater levels of drug-related problems than European Americans (Herd, 1994). It is theorized that African Americans in general, and African-American males in particular, may be at greater risk of substance abuse and drug-related problems than their European-American counterparts due to being hindered in society by the constant bombardment of what Pierce (1970) categorized as "microaggressions." Microaggressions are defined as subtle insults (verbal/nonverbal, visual, or both) directed toward people of color, frequently automatically or unconsciously (Pierce, 1970). In addition Pierce (1974) has indicated that the nature of life in poor urban African-American communities is often characterized by "extreme mundane stress," a situation that can be constant for African-American youth. The persistent long-term exposure to the poor, stressful urban African-American community experience is suggested to condition those exposed to utilize legal and illicit drugs as a mechanism for escape (Pierce, 1974).

Miller, Webster, and MacIntosh (2002) have also attempted to understand the chronic daily stressors urban African-American adolescents face, their reaction to the stressors, and the consequences of the stressors. They utilized the Urban Hassles Scale in their research that was designed to capture the nuances of the African-American urban environment. These findings indicated that daily stressful experiences of urban African-American adolescents might contribute to detrimental outcomes and the development of maladaptive response patterns that could include self-harming behavior.

Substance abuse indirectly influences the risk of suicide for youth because it contributes to chaotic, unstable familial environments that compromise nurturing relationships. These environments contribute to the risk of suicide if the family situation includes issues such as sexual and physical abuse (Hernandez, Lodico, & Diclemente, 1993). In general, difficulties in familial relationships that include abuse, martial discord, and domestic violence increase the risk of suicide (Nisbet, 1996; Summerville, Kaslow, Abbate, & Cronan, 1994; Walter et al., 1995).

Substance abuse is also frequently related to the youth violence that plagues many poverty-ridden urban African-American communities. The disproportionate frequency of illicit drug activity in some African-American urban communities is often accompanied by the youth violence and related contact with the criminal justice system that has a disproportionate negative impact on young African-American male youth (Caetano & Clark, 1998; Hill, 2000; Wade, 1994). Exposure to substance-abuse-related violent behavior appears to be associated with an increased risk for suicide. Pastore, Fisher, and Friedman (1996) reported a doubled likelihood for suicide among adolescents who have experienced violence in their community. This could be a particularly relevant finding given the high levels of exposure to violence present in some poor African-American communities (Mazza & Reynolds, 1999; Richters & Martinez, 1993). The authors will present original research findings in this article that suggest spirituality could contribute to the prevention of suicidal behavior.

SPIRITUALITY AS A PROTECTIVE FACTOR

The rise in suicide rates among youth and the influence of risk factors has contributed to the search for ways to promote protective factors that contribute to resiliency in African-American male youth. Rutter (1987) characterizes resilience as protective mechanisms or processes that are healthy responses to stressful circumstances. The authors of this article believe spirituality and the process of developing spiritual values warrants consideration as a protective factor. There is a scarcity of research on the influence of spirituality as a protective factor. The difficulty of identifying, describing, and quantifying an abstract concept like spirituality is a complex task that appears to encompass ambiguity and subjectivity. The opportunity for ambiguity is heightened by the absence of any coherent language to describe spirituality (Rodger, 1982). However, some theorists and clinicians appear to have made significant contributions toward clarifying of the concept in ways that assist in identifying the protective characteristics of spirituality.

Spirituality is most commonly associated with religion, but it is not synonymous with religion. Contemporary scholars have attempted to clarify various meanings attributed to spirituality and some of these definitions are summarized by Elkins, Hedstrom, Hughes, Leaf, and Saunders (1988) into nine components of spirituality. The nine components include: 1) a transcendent dimension; 2) meaning and purpose in life; 3) mission in life; 4) sacredness of life; 5) material values; 6) altruism; 7) idealism; 8) an awareness of life's tragic and beneficial outcomes; and 9) rewards. Spirituality has also been described as both an individual and communal phenomenon that is not a selfish pursuit and allows individuals to experience passion, creativity, motivation, growth, and change (Chaffers, 1994).

In addition, Mattis (2000) conducted a concept analysis of the written narratives of African-American women that included a characterization of spirituality. This analysis supports a concept of spirituality that includes (a) a belief in a higher power; (b) positively influencing relationships with others; (c) peace, calm and centeredness; as well as (d) efforts to manage adversity through support. Meraviglia (1999) has provided a critical analysis of spirituality, distinguishing it from religiosity. Spirituality was defined as a dynamic integration of mind, body and spirit that reflects a faith in God/ supreme being and a connectedness with oneself, others, nature, or God.

The Afrocentric conceptualization of spirituality includes human connectedness similar to that described by Meraviglia (1999). The values relevant to the Afrocentric paradigm are reflected in the Nguzo Saba, which is Swahili for the 'seven principles' articulated and promoted by Karenga (1996) and other Afrocentric, Africentric, and African-centered scholars as guidelines for living (Azibo, 1996). These seven principles are: 1) unity, 2) self-determination, 3) collective work and responsibility, 4) cooperative economics, 5) purpose, 6) creativity, and 7) faith. Spirituality is a key theme in these principles. The African sense of spirituality was woven into the fabric of society not as a systemized set of religious beliefs or practices but as a central characteristic of the African psyche (Boyd-Franklin, 1989). As it relates to people of African descent, spirituality has in many instances incorporated a conviction about spiritual power and the unquestionable belief that something greater than themselves was watching over them and could provide relief (Brisbane & Womble, 1985).

The absence of spirituality being displayed in one's life and social relationships is proposed to result in a condition of spiritual alienation that could contribute to unhealthy attitudes toward drug use and suicidal behavior. Spiritual alienation is defined as the inability to internalize the spiritual concept of self and others, the inability to acknowledge the importance of a higher power or force, and disproportionate associations of self-worth with materialism (Schiele, 2000). It is further theorized that there is an increased likelihood that individuals with high spiritual alienation will develop unhealthy attitudes toward drug use due to their disconnectedness from self, others, and a higher power or force. These conditions are hypothesized to be prerequisites for suicidal behavior.

THE INFLUENCE OF SPIRITUALITY

Research presented will suggest that spirituality could contribute to the prevention of suicidal behavior. There is some evidence that spirituality as displayed in religious beliefs may buffer many African Americans from the destructive effects that are associated with suicidal behavior (Early, 1992). Research has found that religious African-American youth are more likely than less religious African-American youth to overcome the social and economic handicaps of their inner-city environments (Freeman & Holtzer, 1986). Research findings recently published (Wallace et al., 2003) suggest that religion is an important protective factor helping to prevent young people from engaging in behavior that previous research has found linked to adolescent mortality and morbidity. Conceptually, an Afrocentric perspective on health argues that the more Afrocentric values a young African-American male internalizes, the healthier this individual is, and the more resistant he is to suicidal behavior (Akbar, 1981; Oliver, 1989). This conceptualization suggests that an internalization of an Afrocentric-value-oriented spirituality could provide young African-American males with a protective mechanism that might minimize risk factors related to suicidal behavior. The presence of unhealthy drug attitudes is considered a precursor for drug usage, drug distribution activity, externally directed violence and internally directed violence (suicide). A study by Washington (2003), conducted in one of the poorest neighborhoods of Atlanta, explored the relationships between spirituality and drug attitudes among 61 African-American preadolescent males. The following original report of the findings related to the relationship between spirituality and drug attitudes is part of a larger study on the influence of Afrocentric values. The demographics of this convenience sample are described in Table 1. The study hypothesized that the presence of higher levels of spirituality among

TABLE 1　The Relationships Between Spirituality and Drug Attitudes Study Demographics

	n	Percent
Annual income		
$0–9,999	45	73.7
$10,000–19,999	10	16.4
$20,000–29,999	3	4.9
$30,000–39,999	3	4.9
Number of boys in household		
1	23	37.7
2	24	39.3
3	13	21.3
4	1	1.6
Boy's age		
9	21	34.4
10	13	21.3
11	9	14.8
12	18	29.5
Boy's school grade		
Second	5	8.2
Third	18	29.5
Fourth	10	16.4
Fifth	8	13.1
Sixth	17	27.9
Seventh	3	4.9

the sample would correlate with the presence of higher levels of healthy drug attitudes. Healthy drug attitudes were defined as those against the use of cigarettes, alcohol and illicit drugs.

MEASURING SPIRITUALITY

Measuring spirituality in children is a complex and challenging undertaking. Most of the studies identified in a review of the literature have utilized qualitative research designs. Attempts to quantify an approach for measuring spirituality to allow for statistical manipulation include utilizing the Cultural Questionnaire for Children (CQC). The CQC was designed by Jagers and Owens-Mock (1993) to measure an Afrocultural social ethos that is defined as a combination of spiritual, communal, and affective orientations of people of African descent. The CQC includes three subscales: 1) the Communal Orientation Scale (COS), 2) the Spirituality Orientation Scale (SOS), and 3) the Affective Orientation Scale (AOS). The three subscales measure the presence of communal, spiritual, and/or affective values in African-American children. A unique design feature of each of these three subscales is the utilization of a series of vignettes that describes the attitudes and behavior of the actor. The scales therefore actually question and measure the respondent's perception of congruence between the presence of communal, spiritual, and/or affective values in the actor and himself. Washington (2003) utilized the Communal Orientation Scale (COS) and the Spirituality Orientation Scale (SOS), components of the CQC, in a larger study that investigated the influence of collectivity (communal values) and spirituality on the drug attitudes of black boys. The SOS had one vignette and four items (see Appendix A). The combined scores on items 3 and 4 (score range, 1 to 4) measure spirituality. High scores reflect high levels of spirituality while low scores reflect low levels of spirituality. The Cronbach alpha reliability coefficient of the SOS was .71. This coefficient is considered acceptable for a study of this design. It is also important to note that this is a new instrument that its authors (Mock and Jagers) are still testing.

SPIRITUALITY AND HEALTHY DRUG ATTITUDES

The Pearson *r* correlation coefficient was utilized to measure the relationships between the variable spirituality as measured by the SOS and drug attitudes as measured by the Favorable Attitude Toward Drug Use Scale (FATDUS). The FATDUS was developed by the Center for Substance Abuse Prevention (1993). It includes four items presented in the Likert scale where the scores range from 1 to 4 (see Appendix B). Low scores reflect unhealthy attitudes toward drug use. The Cronbach's reliability coefficient for the FATDUS was .78. This is a stronger degree of reliability than for many similar studies of this nature.

For analysis the Pearson *r* correlation coefficient was utilized. As indicated in Table 2, the resulting correlation test statistic, $r = .217, > .05$, describes modest a statistically significant correlation. Although the correlation coefficient is small or low, there is nevertheless some evidence of a positive relationship (Montcalm & Royse, 2002). The findings of correlation

TABLE 2 Correlations of Collectivity, Spirituality, and Ethnic Identity with Drug Attitudes (N = 61)

		Collectivity	Spirituality	Ethnic identity	Drug attitudes
Collectivity	Pearson correlation	1	.169 .096	**.394 .001	−.074 .573
Spirituality	Pearson correlation	0.169 .096	1	−.012 .464	*.217 .094
Ethnic identity	Pearson correlation	**.394 .001	−.012 .464	1	.075 .568
Drug attitudes	Pearson correlation	−.074 .573	*.217 .047	.075 .568	1

**Correlation is significant at 0.01 level (two tailed).
*Correlation is significant at 0.05 level (one tailed).

for the variable collectivity and ethnic identity in the larger Washington (2003) study with the variable drug attitudes were not statistically significant.

DISCUSSION

This evidence of a relationship between spirituality and drug attitudes among preadolescent African-American males is added to a scarcity of empirical evidence of the potential of spirituality as a protective factor for suicide. There exists a larger body of literature that has attempted to explore and clarify the relationships between religion, substance usage and adolescents (Gorsuch, 1988, 1995; Johnson, Tomkins, & Webb, 2002; Wallace et al., 2003). Studying spirituality as a value or orientation outside the context of religious behavior has not received as much empirical research attention. This is probably due in part to the challenge involved in studying abstract cultural concepts like spirituality. It can also be a challenge to accurately measure the attitudes of youth. The Washington (2003) Atlanta study was designed to follow up on previous research that took on these challenges. Its design as an exploratory analysis of the influence of cultural values (spirituality) and the drug attitudes among "at-risk" young African-American males had methodology limitations that are important to note.

The homogeneous characteristics of the sample, while important for learning about the young people in the sample, limits the generalization of the results to people outside the sample. Also the sample size in the Washington (2003) Atlanta study limits the generalization of the study's findings. Although efforts were taken by the researchers to ensure a valid standardized instrument was utilized as it relates to spirituality, further research is needed to test the reliabilty of the SOS.

A qualitative and quantitative research design maybe most appropriate given the challenges of quantifying such an abstract concept. This is true in part because the dynamic nature of human developmental processes as it relates to abstract concepts such as culture and attitudes can be difficult to measure. If similar sample types are studied, future research designs should also incorporate statistical analysis techniques that better account for the outcome data being skewed in favor of healthy drug attitudes.

Finally, the lack of content analysis of the concept of spirituality in the Washington (2003) Atlanta study restricted knowledge about spirituality as understood by these respondents. Some theorists indicate that while spirituality is difficult to describe, it may be easier to recognize (Copley, 1994; King, 1992; Raitt, 1987). Although it is difficult to describe, it is important to attempt a description because without conceptual limits, definitions of spirituality risk being meaningless (Nye & Hay, 1996). In future research there is a need to systematically explore what concept or understanding of spirituality is being measured. The inclusion of qualitative research approaches that include concept mapping may contribute significantly to the clarification of which definition of spirituality holds the greatest potential for suicide prevention.

IMPLICATIONS

The nature of young African-American male suicide, spirituality, and the findings of the Washington (2003) Atlanta study have implications for suicide-prevention programs that target African-American male youth. There is a need for greater understanding about the fluctuations in the suicide rates of this population and the factors that that influence these rates. The connection between drug use and adolescent mortality is receiving increasing research attention and there continues to be a need for early intervention prevention efforts. Continued development of instruments that measure stressors of urban African-American male youth and potential protective factors such as spirituality could be valuable contributors to the effective design, implementation, and positive outcomes of suicide-prevention programs. The Urban Hassles Scale and the Spirituality Orientation Scale could be valuable tools for examining these stressors, the relationship to self-destructive behavior, and the influence of spirituality upon these stressors and behavior.

The potential for reducing unhealthy drug attitudes via spirituality promotion is encouraging but needs further exploration. It is also important to clarify the possibility that suicide-prevention efforts could be enhanced by incorporating activities that contribute to the development and clarification of spirituality as part of the value system of these youth. Group discussion and interactive approaches that incorporate adult African-American males in the debating of the positive and negative attributes of spirituality might also contribute to the effectiveness of such suicide-prevention approaches.

ACKNOWLEDGEMENT

The authors would like to thank the University of Tennessee College of Social Work for their support of this work.

REFERENCES

Akbar, N. (1981). Mental disorder among African-Americans. *Black Books Bulletin*, 7(2), 18–25.

Azibo, D. A. (Ed.). (1996). *African psychology in historical perspective and related commentary*. Trenton, NJ: Africa World Press.

Bell, C. C. and Clark, D. C. (1998). Adolescent suicide. *Pediatric clinics of North America, 45*, 365–380.

Boyd-Franklin, N. (1989). *Black families in therapy*. New York: Guilford.

Brisbane, F. and Womble, M. (1985–1986). Treatment of black alcoholics. *Alcoholism Treatment Quarterly, 2*(3/4).

Caetano, R. and Clark, C. L. (1998). Trends in drinking patterns among whites, blacks and hispanics: 1984–1995. *Journal of Studies of Alcohol, 54*(3), 659–668.

Centers for Disease Control and Prevention (CDC). (1998). Suicide among black youths–United States, 1980–1995. *Morbidity and Mortality Weekly Report, 47*, 193–196.

Center for Substance Abuse Prevention. (1993). *Drug Attitude Scale*. COPA Project. Rockville, MD: Office of Scientific Analysis.

Chaffers, J. (1994, May 25). *Spirituality – The missing "i" in mass product(i)on: Or why "mass quality" need not be an oxymoron*. Conference proceedings of the Association of Collegiate Schools of Architecture European Conference: The Urban Scene and the History of the Future, London.

Chipungu, S., Hermann, J., Sambrano, S., Nistler, M., Sale, E., and Springer, J. F. (2000). Prevention programming for African American youth: A review of strategies in CSAP'S national cross-site evaluation of high-risk youth programs. *Journal of Black Psychology, 26*(4), 360–385.

Copley, T. (1994). *Religious Education 7–11*. London: Routeledge.

De La Rosa, M. R., Segal, B., and Lopez, R. (Eds.). (1999). *Conducting drug abuse research with minority populations*. New York: Haworth Press.

Early, K. E. (1992). *Religion and suicide in the African American community*. Westport, CT: Greenwood Press.

Elkins, D., Hedstrom, L., Hughes, L., Leaf, J., and Saunders. (1988). Toward a humanistic phenomenological: Definition, description and measurement. *Journal of Humanistic Psychology, 28*, 5–18.

Freeman, R. and Holtzer, H. (Eds.). (1986). *The Black Youth Employment Crisis*. Chicago: University of Chicago Press.

Garland, A. F. and Zigler, E. (1993). Adolescent suicide prevention current research and social policy implications. *American Psychologist, 48*, 169–182.

Gibbs, J. T. (1997). African American suicide: A cultural paradox. *Suicide and Life Threatening Behavior, 27*, 68–79.

Goldsmith, S., Pellmar, T., Kleinman, A., and Bunney, W. (Eds.). (2002). *Reducing suicide: A national imperative*. Committee on Pathophysiology & Prevention of Adolescent & Adult Suicide, Board on Neuroscience and Behavioral Health, Institute of Medicine.

Gorsuch, R. L. (1988). Psychology of religion. *Annual Review of Psychology, 39*, 201–221.

Gorsuch, R. L. (1995). Religious aspects of substance abuse and recovery. *Journal of Social Issues, 51*(2), 65–83.

Herd, D. (1994). Predicting drinking problems among black and white men: Results from a national survey. *Journal of Studies on Alcohol, 55*(1), 61–71.

Hernandez, J. T., Lodico, M., and DiClemente, R. J. (1993). The effects of child abuse and race on risk-taking in male adolescents. *Journal of the National Medical Association, 85*, 593–597.

Hill, R. B. (2000). *Impact of public policy on African-American children*. Annual African-American Families Conference at University of Georgia, Athens, GA.

Jagers, R. J. and Owens-Mock, L. (1993). Culture and social outcomes among inner-city African-American children: An afro-graphic exploration. *Journal of Black Psychology, 19*(4), 391–405.

Johnson, B. R., Tomkins, R. B., and Webb, D. (2002). *Objective hope: Assessing the effectiveness of faith-based organization: A review of the literature* (research report). Philadelphia: Center for Research on Religion and Urban Civil Society, University of Pennsylvania.

Karenga, M. (1996). The nguza saba (The seven principles): Their meaning and message. In M. K. Asante and A. S. Abarry (Eds.), *African intellectual heritage* (pp. 543–554). Philadelphia: Temple University Press.

King, U. (1992). Spirituality, society and culture. *The Way Supplement, 73*, 14–23.

Mattis, J. (2000). African-American women's definitions of spirituality and religiosity. *Journal of Black Psychology, 26*, 101–122.

Mazza, J. J. and Reynolds, W. M. (1999). Exposure to violence in young inner-city adolescents: Relationships with suicidal ideation, depression, and PTSD symptomology. *Journal of Abnormal Child Psychology, 27*, 203–213.

Meraviglia, M. (1999). Critical analysis of spirituality and its empirical indicators: Prayer and meaning in life. *Journal of Holistic Nursing, 17*, 18–33.

Miller, D. B., Webster, S. E., and MacIntosh, R. (2002). What's there and what's not: Measuring daily hassles in urban African American adolescents. *Research on Social Work Practice, 12*(3), 375–3898.

Montcalm, D. and Royse, D. (2002). *Data analysis: For social workers.* Boston: Allyn and Bacon.

Nisbet, P. A. (1996). Protective factors for suicidal black females. *Suicide and Life-Threatening Behavior, 26*, 325–341.

Nye, R. and Hay, D. (1996). Identifying children's spirituality: How do you start without a starting point? *British Journal of Religious Education, 18*(3), 144–154.

Oliver, W. (1989). Black males and social problems: Prevention through Afrocentric socialization. *Journal of Black Studies, 20*(1), 15–39.

Pastore, D. R., Fisher, M., and Friedman, S. B (1996). Violence and mental health problems among urban high school students. *Journal of Adolescent Health, 18*, 320–324.

Pierce, C. (1970). Offensive mechanisms. In F. Barbour (Ed.), *The black seventies* (pp. 265–282). Boston: Peter Sargent.

Pierce, C. (1974). Psychiatric problems of the black minority. In S. Arieti (Ed.), *American handbook of psychiatry* (pp.512–523). New York: Basic Books.

Raitt, J. (1987). Saints and sinners: Roman Catholic and Protestant spirituality in the sixteenth century. In J. Raitt (Ed.), *Christian Spirituality II*. London: RKP.

Reid, J. D., Lee, E. S., Jedlicka, D., and Shin, Y. (1977). Trends in black health. *Phylon, 38*, 105–116.

Rich, C. L., Fowler, R. C., Fogarty, L. A., and Young, D. (1998). San Diego suicide study III: Relationships between diagnoses and stressors. *Archives of General Psychiatry, 45*, 589–592.

Richters, J. E. and Martinez, P. E. (1993). The NIMH community violence project I: Children as victims of and witnesses to violence. *Psychiatry, 56*, 7–21.

Rodger, A. R. (1982). *Education and faith in an open society*. Edinburgh: The Handsel Press.

Rutter, M. (1987). Psychosocial resilience and protective mechanisms. *American Journal of Orthopsychiatry, 57*(3), 316–331.

Schiele, J. H. (2000). *Human services and the afro-centric paradigm*. Binghamton, NY: Haworth Press.

Summerville, M. B., Kaslow, N. J., Abbate, M. E., and Cronan, S. (1994). Psychopathology, family functioning, and cognitive style in urban minority adolescents with suicide attempts. *Journal of Abnormal Child Psychology, 22*, 221–235.

U.S. Department of Health and Human Services. (2002). *2001 National Household Survey on Drug Abuse*. Retrieved June 13, 2002, from: http://www.samhsa.gov/nhsda/2kluhsdal/vol 1/toc.htm#r1

Wade, J. C. (1994). Substance abuse: Implications for counseling African-American men. *Journal of Mental Health Counseling, 16*(4), 415–434.

Wallace, J. M., Brown, T. N., Bachman, J. G., and Laveist, T. A. (2003). The influence of race and religion on abstinence from alcohol, cigarettes and marijuana among adolescents. *Journal of Studies on Alcohol, 64*(6), 843–848.

Walter, H. J., Vaughn, R. D., Armstrong, B., Krakoff, R. Y., Maldonado, L. M., Tiezzi, L. M., and McCarthy, J. F. (1995). Sexual, assaultive, and suicidal behavior among urban minority junior high school students. *Journal of the American Academy of Child and Adolescent Psychiatry, 34*, 73–80.

Washington, G. (2003). *An analysis of the influence of Afrocentric values and the drug attitudes of young African-American males*. Unpublished doctoral dissertation, Clark Atlanta University, Atlanta, GA.

APPENDIX A

CULTURAL QUESTIONNAIRE FOR CHILDREN

Original Spirituality Vignette

Fred believes very strongly in God. He thinks people and all things are made by God and therefore have God in them. Because all things have a spiritual quality, Fred tries to show respect for them instead of thinking of things simply as objects to be used for his own purposes.

1) Fred is _____ most of my friends.

1	2	3	4
not at all like	not much like	somewhat like	very much like

2) Fred is _____ most of my family.

1	2	3	4
not at all like	not much like	somewhat like	very much like

3) Fred is _____ me.

1	2	3	4
not at all like	not much like	somewhat like	very much like

4) How do you feel about Fred?

1	2	3	4
strongly dislike	dislike	like	strongly like

APPENDIX B

FAVORABLE ATTITUDES TOWARD DRUG USE SCALE

DIRECTIONS: PLEASE CAREFULLY READ EACH QUESTION AND CIRCLE YOUR RESPONSE.

1. How wrong do you think it is for someone your age to drink beer, wine, or hard liquor? (For example vodka, whiskey, or gin)

   Very wrong   Wrong   A little bit wrong   Not wrong at all

2. How wrong do you think it is for someone your age to smoke cigarettes?

   Very wrong   Wrong   A little bit wrong   Not wrong at all

3. How wrong do you think it is for someone your age to smoke marijuana?

   Very wrong   Wrong   A little bit wrong   Not wrong at all

4. How wrong do you think it is for someone your age to use LSD, cocaine, amphetamines or another illegal drug?

   Very wrong   Wrong   A little bit wrong   Not wrong at all

3

Acculturative Stress, Violence, and Resilience in the lives of Mexican-American Youth

LORI K. HOLLERAN and SOYON JUNG
University of Texas at Austin, Austin, Texas, USA

This ethnographic study examines the experiences of Mexican American youth in the Southwest, illuminating a number of stressors, traumas, and strengths. It considers the overlay of culture, ethnicity, and experience of stress and violence in personal and interpersonal arenas. While some of these experiences are common to all groups, this article illustrates the perspective of Mexican American youth working out their identities in the midst of their unique stressors including acculturative processes, Mexican families, gangs, and poverty. Phinney (1996, p. 146) defines ethnic identity as the "subjective sense of ethnic group membership." Ethnic minority status has long been considered a stressor for many cultural groups. For Latino/a adolescents many sociocultural experiences related to the acculturation process are often perceived as stressful (Marsiglia, Kulis, & Hecht, 2001). This paper looks at acculturative stress variables as well as traumas including violence, death, abuse, and prejudice.

Social scientists have recognized for over a decade that risk factors and protective factors influence youth outcomes (Cowen & Work, 1988). Clearly, stressors and traumas are risk factors for substance abuse (Hawkins, Catalano, & Miller, 1992). Research has long demonstrated that by focusing on risk and protective factors, negative outcomes can be eliminated, reduced, or mitigated, thus enhancing resiliency (Lorion, Price, & Eaton, 1989).

Ultimately, the youth in this study demonstrate how the stressors and traumas in their lives are reframed and reworked to create strength and buffer risks of negative outcomes. Resilience is influenced by such diverse characteristics as ethnicity, gender, age, sexual orientation, religiosity, and economic status; it is expressed and affected by a variety of systems, including family, school, peers, neighborhood, community, and society (Holleran, Kim, & Dixon, 2004). In addition, it is affected by the availability of environmental resources (Greene & Conrad, 2001). This article explores these young people's experiences in these realms and the ways that the youth integrate perceptions and events into their identities.

ACCULTURATIVE STRESS AMONG MEXICAN-AMERICAN ADOLESCENTS OF THE SOUTHWEST

Anthropologists Redfield, Linton, and Herskovists (1936) define acculturation as "phenomena which result when groups of individuals having different cultures come into continuous first-hand contact, with subsequent changes in the original culture patterns of either or both groups" (p. 149). At individual level, acculturation, which is often specified as "psychological acculturation," involves changes in numerous aspects of an individual including attitudes, behaviors, beliefs, and values, as a consequence of acculturation (Wong, 1999). Acculturation often causes inevitable stress and acculturative stress could be serious when social norms and values of the dominant culture are in conflict with those of the culture of origin (Gilbert & Cervantes, 1986). Stressors in acculturation process encompass communication difficulties, divergent value systems, psychological challenges, prejudice, and various social stressors (Berry & Kim, 1988).

Acculturation affects Mexican-American adolescents of the borderlands perhaps more than any other population. Because of the proximity to the motherland of Mexico and the porous nature of the imposed geographic boundary, the adolescents may experience greater tensions related to loyalty than other groups. Stavans (1995) describes the tension of the borderlands as "a never-never land near the rim and ragged edge we call frontier, an uncertain, indeterminate, adjacent area that everybody can recognize and that, more than ever before, many call our home" (p. 17).

The tension between the two cultures exists in all the facets of the lives of Mexican-American youth. Within family, often there is a wide gap between parents, the first generation migrants, and their U.S.-born children in terms of familiar languages and their weltanschauung that make parent-child communication difficult. In addition, Mexican-American parents may vicariously attempt to have their dreams and ambitions fulfilled by their children. The children may feel such parental attempts as pressure (Suárez-Orozco & Suárez-Orozco, 1995). Another burden for Mexican-American adolescents is that they are supposed to take various family responsibilities such as translating, acting as buffers between the family and the new culture, sibling care, and the like (Taylor, Hurley, & Riley, 1986). These are not the typical expected roles for adolescents from non-immigrant families.

Mexican American youth are also exposed to other types of stressors in social contexts. At school they often undergo racial-ethnic prejudice of classmates and school personnel fail to support and value them (Galguera, 1998; Suárez-Orozco, 1989; Suárez-Orozco, & Suárez-Orozco, 1995). Moreover, second and subsequent generations of migrants may experience a sense of deprivation and marginality vis-à-vis the majority culture (Horowitz, 1983; Suárez-Orozco and Suárez-Orozco, 1995) because their aspirations are more likely to go unrealized compared to those from dominant culture (Rogler, Cortes, & Malgady, 1991).

It is well documented that stress is significantly related to various mental health problems such as depression (Avison & McAlpine, 1992; D'Arcy & Siddique, 1984), and alcohol and drug use among adolescents in general, and minority adolescents in particular (Alva, 1995; Bry, McKeon, & Pandina, 1982; Feliz-Ortiz, & Newcomb, 1992). Although there is further need for exploration, several previous studies reported a significant association between acculturative stress and substance use and abuse. According to Vega, Zimmerman, Warheit, and Gill (1995), for example, acculturative stress reported by adolescents was positively linked to early drug experimentation, family drug use, and per drug use. Similarly, in a study on Hispanic adolescents (Alva, 1995), stress related to intergroup conflicts, communication problems, and peer relations, much of which overlap with the construct of acculturative stress, differentiate alcohol users and nonusers among Hispanic adolescents.

VIOLENCE EXPERIENCE: TRAUMA OF MEXICAN AMERICAN IMMIGRANTS

Colonialism implies virtual genocide to Mexicans. They were robbed of land titles, professionally disregarded, used as commodities, and viewed as inferior beings in relation to language, ritual, and religious traditions (Vélez-Ibáñez, 1996). Vélez-Ibáñez (1996) identifies a number of historical antecedents to cultural subordination of Mexicans as follows: 1) the rise of Anglo commercial activities; 2) the destructive effects of the illegal arms trade which devastated populations, the economy, and social structures; 3) the Texas War of Independence in 1836; 4) the Mexican War of 1846; 5) the invasion of intensive capitalist enterprises resulting in stratified class communities; and 6) the institutional subordination in employment (e.g., dual wages for the same jobs in favor of whites), education, politics, economy, and even recreation.

The influences of these traumatic experiences appear to remain in the current lives of Mexicans and Mexican Americans. First of all, internalized colonialism is a powerful force with which to be reckoned. As Freire (1993) notes, the oppressed are at the same time the oppressor as a result of internalized colonialism. This perspective helps to explain how many of the U.S.-born Mexican Americans are not very respectful to recent Mexican immigrants, even though they have the same ethnic background.

Furthermore, many Mexican Americans are still exposed to and threatened by violence in their daily lives. Previous studies have reported higher prevalence rates of Hispanics compared to their white counterparts in numerous violence-related incidents or victimization including sexual victimization (Kercher & McShane, 1984), adolescent weapon carrying (Carvajal, Hanson, Romero, & Coyle, 2002), violent offending (Perez, 2001), and injury due to physical fight and (Centers for Disease Control and Prevention, 1996).

Obviously, exposure to and experience of violence contribute to various negative psychological outcomes and social relation problems. According to Perez (2001), the experience of physical and sexual abuse as a child is significantly associated with self-reported delinquency in adolescence such as property, violent, and sex offenses. In general these effects sustained even after academic performance, family structure, and economic deprivation were taken into account (Perez, 2001). It is also noteworthy that teenagers who regarded gangs, strangers, and racial tension as stressors are more likely to smoke cigarettes, drink alcohol and use marijuana (Allison, Adlaf, & Tates, 1997).

STRENGTH PERSPECTIVE & RESILIENCE OF MEXICAN AMERICAN YOUTH

Previous literature tends to interpret Mexican American culture from a deficit-focused perspectives (Aguirre & Baker, 2000). These perspectives devalue traditional Mexican-American culture on the grounds that traditional norms interfere with assimilation of Mexican immigrants to American society (Holleran & Waller, 2003). This implies that assimilation—acculturation achieved by abandoning original cultural heritages and by adopting those of a new culture—is viewed as desirable in a deficit-focused perspective. During the past 20 years, however, numerous scholars have indicated the limitations of deficit-focused perspectives. First of all, it is noted that Mexican Americans who try to assimilate are more vulnerable to psychological distress, when compared with those who maintain strong bonds to their original culture (Burnam, Hough, Karno, Escobar, & Teller, 1987; Falicov, 1996; Ortiz & Arce, 1984; Warheit, Veta, Auth, & Meinhardt, 1985). In addition, Hispanic adolescents were found to be more resilient, when compared with their white peers, to uncontrollable stressors and parental alcoholism (Barrera, Li, & Chassin, 1993, 1995). The strength and availability of Hispanic social supports was presented as a major probable explanation for such resilience (Barrera & Reese, 1993).

Contrary to the assimilation stance, a social adaptation perspective regards adherence to the traditional values and beliefs as beneficial. Strong ties to one's own ethnic culture is viewed as a source of strength that allows individuals and groups to adapt and maintain "resilience, flexibility, and cohesion in the face of changing social environments and economic circumstances" (Berardo, 1991, p. 6). In this point of view, culture is metaphorically described as "the roots that sustain and nourish a plant" (Falicov, 1996, p. 170) because culture upholds and nurtures human beings. This view is harmoniously matched with the strengths perspective (Saleebey, 1997), which values culture as the fundamental foundation for identity and as a reservoir of resources for smooth adaptation and successful coping.

Another crucial common ground of social adaptation and the strength perspective is the emphasis on resilience. Resilience refers to positive adaptations despite the presence of adversity (Waller, 2001). Adversity is often indexed with risk factors, which cause or aggravate undesirable outcomes such as alcoholism, drug abuse, delinquency, and teen pregnancy (Jessor, 1993). In contrast, protective factors are considered to facilitate or augment desirable outcomes by buffering the impacts of adverse environments. It is important to note that proper combination of protective factors might offset the negative impact of risk factors. Given prevalent risk factors such as social challenges and economic deprivation among Mexican Americans, therefore, a primary task should be to seek sources of resilience or protective factors based on social adaptation, as well as a strength perspective (Holleran & Waller, 2003).

METHODOLOGY

Research Design

While some techniques proposed and enlisted by positivist and post-positivist grounded theorists (e.g., theoretical sampling and systematic coding) were utilized, the research design of this study was intentionally emergent and was not bound by the specific set of steps which are viewed by grounded theorists as essential. Though the following research design was predetermined, the researchers and team were ready to adjust and be flexible regarding schedules, observations and interviews, even settings. The naturalistic research is based on the method of ethnography (Vidich & Lyman, 1994). This study's ethnographic research is naturalistic and based on participant observational fieldwork and interpretations of observed data. The research methodology consists of 1) conceptualization and preparation for the study; 2) intensive participant observation in the field setting; 3) data collection through informal contacts, semi-structured interviews, and focus groups; and 4) analytic reflection on the data. The process was not linear; information gathering processes and directions were reevaluated throughout the research via weekly interdisciplinary team meetings and electronic mail notes and memos.

The Sample

The city in which this study took place is one of the most rapidly growing cities in the U.S. with a high concentration of Mexican Americans and African Americans. To have a sample which reflected the internal diversity of Mexican Americans, this study employed theoretical or purposive, rather than random, sampling models (Glaser & Strauss, 1967, Denzin & Lincoln, 1994). High-school and community-center demographics were collected and reviewed. The result was the choice of two community centers and one high school with a large population of Latino/Latina adolescents. The settings also evidenced interactions between the Mexican-American youth and youth of other ethnicities, as well as adults and family members. Participant observation was conducted at all three sites and youths were observed in their natural settings. The group of participants consisted of Mexican Americans from an urban setting with low socioeconomic status. While much of the research on Mexican Americans is done with students, this study consists of both students and dropouts. A total of thirty youths (English speaking and/or bilingual) participated as informants through focus groups and interviews. Eleven Mexican Americans were interviewed individually, nineteen participated in the focus groups, and seven contributed actively to the focus-group processes (i.e., twelve were present but only minimally contributed to the group interview). This yielded a total of eighteen core participants. Eight of the core participants were male; ten were female. The ages of the core participants ranged from 13–18 years old. All but three of these participants were still in school. Nine of the students were from the high-school, and nine were from community centers.

Data Analysis

Data analysis began simultaneously with data collection during the weekly team meetings. The ethnographers' journals, memos, lists of questions, and field notes were reviewed and synthesized during the actual research period. The findings informed the ongoing inquiries and observations of the ethnographers. After the study, the primary author obtained the transcriptions of the focus groups and interviews and conducted both hand and computer analyses on the data. The primary researcher participated in the initial analysis process, which was ongoing through the period of research as well as the analyses of the transcribed data. Secondary analysis was conducted on the interviews and focus groups of all three ethnographers. The analysis of the transcribed data involved the process of coding to elicit patterns and themes in the data. Codes were created, broken into subcategories reflecting the participants' conditions, interactions, strategies, consequences, and styles, and synthesized into themes (Lofland & Lofland, 1995; Strauss, 1987).

FINDINGS

The analyses of the data suggested that Mexican-American youth in the Southwest experience various acculturative stressors and often face traumatic violence. Despite the disadvantageous environments and life experiences, however, these youth, in general, did not display serious problems including substance use/abuse. Furthermore, most of those who were previously involved in serious problem behaviors, such as gang activity, reported that they no longer participated in such antisocial behaviors. This might imply that there is some protective mechanism that augments the resilience of Mexican-American youth. This study explores the sources of resilience among Mexican-American youth along with examining acculturative stressors and the experience of violence in the lives of these adolescents.

Acculturative Stress

Because of the proximity to Mexico and the porous nature of the imposed geographic boundary, acculturation affects adolescent Mexican-American adolescents in the borderlands perhaps more than any other population. They are confronted with tensions that arise from moving between family and Americanized peers, between English and Spanish languages, and between traditional values and those connected with popular American youth culture. In such a situation, the primary tasks of many Mexican-American youth are to adapt themselves to the dominant culture and to maintain a sense of ethnic identity at the same time. Yet, this dual task is not easy to carry out and many of these young people experience substantial stress in the acculturation process. Some of the youth fully embrace the dominant culture and reject their cultures of origin. Others stay intricately tied to their heritage and do not take on the values, practices, and mores of the dominant culture. Still others are marginalized and reject both arenas for alternative cultures. There are many variations on acculturative styles (Berry, 1980; Cuellar & Arnold, 1995; Oetting & Beauvais, 1991) and each encompasses its own stressors.

CRITICISM TOWARD MEXICAN-AMERICAN YOUTH FROM THEIR ETHNIC CULTURE

Most Mexican-American youth are exposed to dominant American culture and educated within the U.S. educational systems. Naturally, they absorb American values and have a good command of English. The acculturative stress that the more acculturated or "Americanized" Mexican-American adolescents frequently face is the criticism that they abandon their ethnic roots and are not good enough to be "a true Mexican." Such criticism becomes particularly salient when the youth are not fluent in Spanish. Carmen added a vignette about this as follows:

> Oh, it's like my grandma will be talking to me in Spanish, ". . . .Ella dice, tu no tiences una lengua mexicana." She goes, "You don't have a tongue of a Mexican," and I be like, "Yes, I do! It just needs practice."

Carmen also shared a stressful experience regarding the use of Spanish at work.

> At my work, this lady, she put me down. She was like, "You're a poor excuse for a Mexican, you don't know Spanish." I was like, "Wow." I go, "It's not my fault.". . . .Just because I'm Mexican, It's like you must speak Spanish.

More assimilated or acculturated U.S.-born Mexican-American youth are also condemned by their peers, especially those from recent immigrant Mexican families. Mark states:

> Because I know Spanish fluent, and I would talk to some of them (white people) and I would get called a "sell out" by the people born in Mexico, they would say, 'you are a sell out.' They say, 'See, you know how to speak Spanish but you don't talk to us.' I said, 'No, it's not like that, I have friends. You know, my mom, that is, all I talk at home is Spanish, so you know you have no right to call me a sell out.'

SCHISM BETWEEN UPWARD MOBILITY AND LOYALTY TO THEIR ETHNIC CULTURE

Criticism for losing the cultural heritage of their ethnic group or high expectation to keep traditional culture might suggest that there is great pressure on Mexican-

American youth not to stretch themselves beyond the ethnic group and be successful in the dominant culture. Mark's story clearly shows this pressure.

> You know, a lot of people, if I talk with real good vocabulary, they are like uh, you know, a lot of them think we are trying to be White actually.

That is, Mexican-American youth appear to encounter what a number of social scientists describe as a schism between "upward mobility" or the "American dream" and "honor" or "loyalty" regarding ethnic priorities (Horowitz, 1983; Romanucci-Ross & De Vos, 1995).

TENSION BETWEEN U.S.-BORN ENGLISH-SPEAKING MEXICAN-AMERICAN ADOLESCENTS AND MEXICAN-BORN SPANISH-SPEAKING ADOLESCENTS

To make matters worse, it is not rare that U.S.-born Mexican-American youth accept dominant American culture without question and exhibit internalized colonialism. These youth view recent Mexican immigrants from the Americanized standpoint rather than their traditional ethnic perspective. For example, some informants characterized less-acculturated Mexican immigrants as "welfare-dependent" or "starting and not finishing things," alluding to the informants' Americanized values:

> Mundo: Well, um, well, that's my own opinion of them. I think they're (wetback)'re nosey. I think they're always, like, they always, how would I say? They're the type that, um, start something, but can't finish it.

More notably, informants often used the pejorative term 'wetback' to indicate Spanish-speaking, less-acculturated Mexicans. Marla's description about 'wetbacks' shows a negative perspective against recent Mexican immigrants even more clearly:

> Marla: To me, it's [Mexico] so dirty and ugly, dirty and ugly (laughs) and the people stink (laughs more heartily).
> Interviewer: In Mexico?
> Marla: Well, in our part, like wetbacks, I mean.
> Interviewer: What part is that?
> Marla: It's like um, it's in Juarez, it's called Juarez, Mexico. Well, usually the people, like some of the Mexicans like kind of clean-cut, wear cowboy hats and the big old belt buckles. They look dumb, but at least they're clean, they keep themselves clean. But in the part that my dad is from, they just run around dirty and don't use deodorant or nothing.
> Interviewer: So if you had to describe a 'wetback' how would you?
> Marla: A person that's real dirty, nasty, goes and messes with young girls and goes with their lips, "chsp, chsp, hey, hey" like that, that to me is a wetback, that's not a Mexican.

> Interviewer: What about the women wetbacks?
> Marla: Um, she's just poppin' out kids here and there just to use the money, like welfare, food stamps and all that. That's what a wetback means.

Although many U.S.-born Mexican-American adolescents appear to utilize assimilation strategies to accomplish acculturative tasks and cope with relevant stress, it is not always appropriate or effective. Assimilation in general and internally colonized attitudes in particular inevitably acerbate the tension between monolingual Spanish-speaking Mexicans and more acculturated, English-speaking Mexican Americans, which could be a serious obstacle to mutual understanding.

> Mark: The wetbacks, what people call, they didn't really hang around the Chicanos or the White people, just around with themselves you know. I mean they didn't really interact.
> Mundo: We don't get along with them, because we think they're different. Why is because like to us, well, my own opinion is that wetbacks, well, them people, they're nosey, they talk too much, you know, I mean, they just don't know where we're coming from, you know.

Mark also describes:

> I mean like what I've heard about the school I'm going to, the Mexicans segregate themselves from the Chicanos and they, I guess, the Chicanos call them 'wetbacks' and stuff, you know, I guess that is the term they use. It's not, I mean, it might be, but I guess, I think it is on both parts, the Chicanos and Mexicans, they are scared to talk to each other. For one, a lot of Mexicans don't speak fluent English and the other is that sometimes Chicanos have a little bit of an attitude.

PREJUDICE AND STEREOTYPES AGAINST ALL MEXICAN-AMERICANS IN U.S. SOCIETY

Another serious stressor that Mexican-American youth suffer is the stereotypes and prejudice against their ethnic group on the whole. Although U.S.-born Mexican-American youth try to make a clear distinction between themselves and recent immigrants, as described above, the two are usually considered the same by American society. Most U.S.-born Mexican-American youth, even though they refer to themselves as Mexicans, vehemently defend against being confused with Mexican-born immigrants. For example, Danny describes a fight that occurred because U.S.-born Mexican-Americans were called 'wetbacks':

> One time, at the school, a stoner got bad with a whole bunch of Mexicans, because there is a lot of Mexicans there, you know, and Blacks, and he got bad. You know, he thought he was all bad and tough, he took off his shirt, "Like what's up, I'll take all of you wetbacks," so they got mad because some of them weren't, you know, so they got

mad and so they just rushed him and jumped him and got his other friends and just beating him up and stuff.

Similarly, Rosie and Wardo both note being upset that people call them 'wetbacks':

> Rosie: The really bad thing is that no matter what, whether you speak Spanish or not, like the Black people, they always call us 'wetbacks.' Because that's just something they call us, but I don't really get into that. That's just ignorant.
> Wardo: A lot of people call us wetbacks and it's like we're not that, so why are you callin' us that? I guess the offensive thing, too, is 'spics' they call us.
> Interviewer: Who would call you that?

Wardo: Like Black people mostly, and like Whites. There might be a couple, but not too often, and even like Mexicans might say, "You're a 'wetback'" and then you'd get mad and be like, "F— you. I ain't from there. What's up?" And a lot of people like play around, but even when you play around with somebody, like when you bump into somebody, they get all mad. Even if you say, "I'm sorry," they say, "I don't give a f—, I'm gonna stick you" or whatever. A lot of stuff happens like that.

Trauma: Experience of Violence & Observation of Death

Aggression and violence are recurrent themes emerging from the data. Violence as well as acculturative stress seems prevalent in the daily lives of Mexican-American youth. Even traumatic incidents involving violence are not uncommon. The informants experienced violence in various places and situations including their homes and social gatherings with peers.

VIOLENCE WITHIN THE FAMILY CONTEXT

Children and adolescents in immigrant families are particularly vulnerable to violence within the family context. With the undercurrent of acculturative stress, such families are prone to family conflicts and violence. The informants in this study were often critical toward their fathers when they perceived they did not fulfill their traditional male role as providers, maltreated their wives, or were indifferent to nurturing children and/or assuming household chores. They connected their critical views of some fathers as providers with their need to be financially independent. Rosita described:

> It's hard, because my dad, he don't have nothing. He's just lying around the house. He says he cleans. He does outside a little, but not all that he says. I have to clean, and help raise the kids. Now it's getting to where I

have to buy my own food. I don't really eat. And like my boyfriend used to feed me. I don't know. I just need to depend on myself right now. I'm supporting myself. I'm trying to get myself out of high school. I'm trying to get myself a car, go to college. I'm doing everything on my own and I'm proud of myself because of what I'm doing.

Apparently, there are structural limitations to the Mexican-American parents' abilities to provide a supportive home environment and enough financial support for their children. A number of the informants' fathers did not have jobs, many lacked the education or training needed for employment beyond the minimum wage, and some of the fathers were entrenched in the cycle of going in and out of jail. Although these fathers failed to fulfill the traditional provider role, some attempted to maintain their influence in the family. This disjunction stripped them from the traditional family power hierarchy. In the situations where traditional parental roles are made obsolete, some fathers used physical power to compensate for the moral power they were losing over their daughters, and the more acculturated daughters were often defiant to such trials. Cristina provides an example:

I used to get physically abused by my dad. But that quit happening because I had told him how I felt about it and I didn't like getting hit so. Like as a girl, I got punched in my face. But I told him how I felt; I just hated getting treated bad and you know, I'm supposed to be respected as a girl.

Sometimes Mexican-American youth justified violence as a measure to protect their family members, reflecting their vulnerable status in the U.S., on the one hand, and their family-oriented, traditional values, on the other. This data illustrates that violent thoughts or actions are often rooted, or at least understood by the informants, in terms of virtues such as protection, loyalty, responsibility, integrity, and kinship. For example, Rosie describes the acts of violence and revenge that resulted from family protectiveness:

If somebody beat up one of my brothers and we know who it is, my brother and my dad and my brother's friends might get together to like find those people... That happened once to my cousin. She was just walking down the street and somebody just threw a bottle or something at her head and she was like, it was like bad. Some of my cousins found out who it was and they went to get them. It turned out to be a few kids from [our rival gang].

VIOLENCE WITHIN PEER CONTEXT

Some of the informants acknowledge that the violence is sought after and even expected in many everyday realms with peers. Due to a lack of structural motivators, such as high academic achievement at school, the need for challenge is channeled into violent interactions. Violence offers the opportunity for heroism through risk. For example, when asked if there are conflicts at parties, Mundo answered:

> At every party...actually that's what people come for. Actually, I've heard my friends say that's what they throw parties for. To have people come, and if there's somebody they don't like they can start stuff. But like, you know, it's our party so we do what we want. But, we're prepared before something happens, so whatever, and like I say, it's bad, but like if someone were to pull out a gun, you know...

As evidenced by his increased energy and animation about the subject, Mundo proudly described the rites of blood:

> [Fights and riots] usually end in somebody getting hurt, somebody dying, somebody becomes disabled or something. It's never going to be solved by talking... our first reaction is we want to fight.

Some of the informants participate in the violence but fear or regret the loss of life. For example, Wardo speaks to the prodigality of life.

> All these people getting killed, it's like, I don't know. Like back when I was in a gang, I was never into killing people or nothing, maybe fighting and stuff, but killing is too far for me.... I've seen a lot of that. Shooting and all that. People shooting at me, and stuff, it ain't fun at all.

OBSERVATION OF DEATH & SUICIDE

The data clearly illustrates that most of the adolescents in the study had witnessed death face-to-face. In the narratives, every day has potential to be a 'Dia de Los Muertos.' Wardo shared his account of watching a friend die:

> I've seen people die. And it's *scary*, like when I saw my friend die in front of my face, it's like seeing my own family die and stuff. That's hard. (pause.) It's like you can't believe it or something. It's like they're sleeping and you try to wake 'em up. It just don't happen. They don't wake up.

Not surprisingly, observing death and loss of loved ones caused extreme reactions in the informants in this study. These experiences were often described as the most shocking event in their lives. For example, Wardo's depiction of his best friend's suicide evidences his confusing and overwhelming feelings. As will be addressed later, Wardo explained this incident was a decisive turning point in his life to stop gang-banging.

Wardo: I used to live with my best friend and that's who I hung around. I used to live with him for a long time too.

Interviewer: What was he like?

Wardo: He was real nice. He was like my brother. But, I don't know, we were just kickin' and like, eventually he died. He committed suicide.

Interviewer: (Sadly) Oh?

Wardo: So that was like a big thing. Like ever since he died, that was it. I changed my whole life. After him, because, to me he was even closer than my brother was, 'cause we did everything together, like anything. Whatever he needed I tried to get it for him and whatever I needed he'd help me.... We were there one time, we were like at a party. For some reason, we were all like having a good time and then he was inside the house with a bunch of friends. And like a lot of people now-a-days they have guns, you know, teenagers, and they have it like, you know, for protection, but I don't know, for some reason, he just, I don't know. No one knows. It's like a mystery why he did it. He told me everything. We used to tell each other everything, like even we used to talk about if we would die, who we would want at our funeral, we used to talk about stuff like that. We always used to tell each other what was on our mind, like if anything was wrong. But he never told me nothing, that's why, it keeps me wondering every day. Why'd he do it?"

Sources of Resilience among Mexican-American Youth

As illustrated previously, acculturative stress and traumatic incidents involving violence are prevalent in the lives of Mexican-American youth. Given previous research reporting the significant relationship between problem behaviors including substance use and acculturative stress as well as traumatic experiences (Allison et al., 1997; Alva, 1995; Perez, 2001; Vega et al., 1995), one of the most notable findings in this study is that most of the 30 participants had not been involved in seriously problematic activities. Even those who had been involved in gang activities no longer displayed serious problems growing. The suggesting that a strong, positive ethnic identity, ethnic pride, and appreciation of and growing up with traditional Mexican values and beliefs such as *familismo* may be protective factors contributing to resilience in Mexican-American adolescents.

ETHNIC IDENTITY AND PRIDE

Throughout history, Mexican Americans have had to fight for and defend their territory, and this experience has served as a metaphor for claiming identity. The claiming and defending of territories (e.g., streets, neighborhoods, and school bleachers) and setting clear boundaries between racial/ethnic groups are major themes in the data. The informants rarely questioned the dynamics around the defense of the established boundaries. Mundo described this phenomenon as follows:

> It's crazy how everybody has their own space. It's like if one group walks into another group's area, it's disrespect. That's how riots start.... That's their territory. It's like crazy how we do it, but it's just like, anybody can walk through it; it's nobody's street, but I mean that's how we go by, it's disrespective [*sic*] and that's exactly how it is in school. We have our own little areas where we kick back, and if another group passes you or whatever, that's disrespect to us.

The general concept about territories and boundaries that Mexican-American youth establish expands to a specific concept about racial-ethnic boundaries. Mexican-American adolescents' perceptions about ethnic boundaries seem distinctive, especially in settings where the diverse racial-ethnic groups coexist, such as school. Rosie figuratively illustrated where Mexicans are at school, distinguishing themselves from other racial-ethnic groups:

> I mean for most people, if you're Mexican, most of your friends are Mexican, and if you're Black, most of your friends are Black. And it's the same for like the places you hang. Like on the quad at school. Right here in the corner, there's Blacks. And like here in the middle, there's Mexicans, and on the other side, there's Whites, who are mostly at the tables studying and stuff.

In addition to ethnic identity, ethnic pride characterizes Mexican-American adolescents. In general, they demonstrate deep pride in their ethnic origin and cultural background. While explaining the difference between Mexican Americans and recent Mexican immigrants, Marla revealed her pride about being a Mexican American:

> Marla: Being proud of your own culture and stuff but not taking it for granted, like saying, 'yeah, I'm from Mexico.' Saying all that and then living off the government here, like it's kind of hard to explain. You can be Mexican and be proud and everything but don't take it for granted, like show it off, just be clean.
> Interviewer: What do you mean by 'show it off'?
> Marla: Usually they all are like shouting out their windows, 'Viva, Mexico!' and this and that. That don't make no sense, they're screaming out Mexico, but they're here. They'll be proud of it, but yet they're not over there because like this government don't care over there and they're over here to use food stamps and stuff like that, at least the women are.

Rosita also stated that she was happy about her ethnic background. Her pride was particularly prominent in terms of Mexican traditional cultural practices.

> I am happy that I'm Mexican... I like cultural things, like Mexican danc-
> ing, I even took Mexican dancing lessons like in 8th grade. But I like the
> food and the Mexican holidays.
>   I like cruising. ... even though others do it, like blacks and whites and
> all, it's mostly a Mexican thing. ... That's like our culture and people have
> been cruising[1] down here for so many years, for like 30 to 40 years. They
> were cruising down Central, and now that it's against the law, it's like part
> of the culture has been taken away. It's bad.

FAMILISMO

Throughout the interviews, the informants consistently expressed their value
of family. Statements emphasizing the importance of family such as "Family
always comes before your homies" and "Trust family more than friends"
were repeated. Monica's description about the relationships, role division,
and collaboration within her family clearly demonstrates '*familismo,*' which
signifies family closeness and loyalty.

> I knew they [her parents] had to take care of...my [younger] brothers and
> sisters. I think that's how me and my two older brothers were. We all
> started working and we did anything just to get money.

Strong mental connection between the informants and their families
supports the previous research findings (Mirandé, 1985) that identify family
as the source of support and comfort in an otherwise unfavorable environment, like a symbolic oasis. To the question, "Where do you feel safe and
why?" Mike answered:

> Probably anywhere with my friends or like if I walk in my neighborhood
> at night... and my house because, I don't know, I guess because I am
> around my family and I feel comfortable around them.

Interestingly, Mike equated safety with comfort level, and his answer
implied that emotional comfort could be attained by family bonding and close
connection among family members. The same theme emerged from stories
about school and interactions with non-Mexican American classmates. Teresa
expressed uncomfortable feelings outside the safe zone of home and barrio:

---

[1]Cruising is a culturally-based tradition which enables Chicanos and Chicanas to spend
time together, explore territories, and display pride in being Mexican American (Hunt, Joe,
& Waldorf, 1996; Rodriguez, 2000). The informants describe taking their cars, which they shine
and adorn, dress up, and drive up and down major roads downtown. While the word cruise at
times is associated with "joy riding," there are a number of factors that have made this action
much more multidimensional in the lives of the youth. For example, cruising means stepping
outside of the familiar territory, often being exposed to violence and tensions. Outside of their
own homes and neighborhoods they described how this expression of culture is scrutinized
and regulated.

I get judged real quick [in school]. When I go home, I don't. I'm not a mean person, I don't know if you guys think I look mean.... Ever since I was in grade school, I have been judged on my appearance. And I don't do that now, judge people by their appearance.

The sense of *familismo* among Mexican-American adolescents did not seem to totally disappear even when their family members were considered undesirable or disloyal to the other family members. Mundo described his unsatisfactory relationship:

I didn't like the way he treated me. He always told me he hated me. He thought that I was like competing with him. He actually told me that my mother loved me more than she loved him. What do you expect? I'm her son."

At the same time, however, Mundo articulated his natural bonding and intent to be loyal to his father. This is clearly revealed in his statements, "I like him" [his father] and "I still have to live up to that I have his name—Mundo."

FOCUSING ON THE POSITIVE

Much of the data revolves around the participants' existential views of life and death. Although the informants were immersed in a world of violence and death, they maintained positive attitudes on life, and meaningful responses to loss, as well as to hopes, plans, and dreams for the future.

Sometimes the informants complained that their circumstance did not satisfy their material needs, but the informants' attitudes about their life situations were, in general, positive. Notably, the informants tried to reframe hardship into strength. Mark shared his positive view of hardship during the interview:

I wouldn't have liked to have grown up in any other place, because, I mean, you learn to value things more if you don't have too much, you know. That's why I think it was pretty good.

Furthermore, informants often regarded suffering and disappointment as something beneficial, as well as an ordinary part of life. This spiritual aspect pervades this study. As described by Olmos, Ybarra, and Monterrey (1999, p. 20), "If even God suffered the crucifixion for us, there must be something good in suffering." In these situations, there is often direct reference to "God" or "the Lord" or "miracles." For example, Mundo prides himself in recuperating from a potentially crippling, near-fatal accident.

Mundo: The thing that I didn't like about my childhood was when I got hit by a car, because they said that I was never going to walk again.

Interviewer: Oh, my...

Mundo: They said they didn't know if I was ever going to walk again and that kinda like messed me up because like now that I'm old enough and active and everything, it's like I can't do all the things that other people can do.... It was like a highlight, being on the news and everything, but still, you know. They could've really messed me up, and it was on my cousin Kristy's birthday... that crazy drunk driver! ...Actually the good thing about it was Christmas Day, actually was the day I learned how to walk. Christmas Day! I tell everybody that—I thought it was a gift from God. Christmas Day I learned how to walk. 'Cause the day before that, Christmas Eve, was when I got my cast taken off and they didn't know if I'd know how to walk and they put me through those bars, you know, where you learn how to walk and I couldn't do it and that Christmas morning I had it, and I like had my crutches and I had someone hold me by the shirt and the next thing I knew I was walking. I thought they were still holding me, but I was walking by myself. And I don't know why, but I just let go of my crutches and I was walking. In just a matter of days! Days!

Ultimately, positive attitudes toward life and the world among Mexican-American youth is also found in their perspective toward violence and gang activity. The informants viewed the presence of violence in their lives as a necessary part of becoming an adult in the community. One youth noted, "I think it's like a cycle of growing up." This concept of necessary suffering, that reflects the concept of *fatalismo*, was common among the informants, implying that these youth accept gang involvement and the experience of violence as somewhat unavoidable and transformative. This might be the key to understanding how and why Mexican-American youth suddenly change the direction of their life paths at a certain juncture in their lives. Denny says:

I want to start turning my life around and start serving the Lord and start going to church and stuff. That way is for a person to be married you know. I know I messed up at first, you know, 'cause marriage first and then do what you gotta do, you know make love, but that came first, so
...before this started I use [sic] to think wrong about things, you know—joined a gang and stuff, and most likely I realized that it's not worth it, it's not worth losing your life for. So one day I seen so many things that most people wouldn't want to see... it's not worth losing your life over a street that I'm never going to own, or never going to have, or take over and stuff. I just decided that I was going to change my life, you know, around. You know, getting back on track... I want to start changing my life around.

It should be noted also that traumatic experiences such as the death of a close friend often lead Mexican-American youth to positive changes, rather than cause mental-health problems such as depression or Posttraumatic

Stress Disorder (PTSD). Specifically, the traumatic experiences seem to awaken Mexican-American youth to the possible result of their disruptive behaviors and inspire them to alter their life courses. It may sound ironic that traumatic experiences have desirable influences on youth. On the basis of their deeply positive attitudes toward life, however, it was the case for some of the informants in this study. In response to the question of how his best friend's suicide changed his life, Wardo responded:

> I just made a big change. That's when I got my job. I just quit going out and like getting in trouble... once he was gone I just left all that behind. I used to hang around with the gang, but I just left all that behind and I came by my Grandma and now I just kick it with my cousins—I just stay with my family now.

Mundo provided another similar example. After observing the death of Nick's brother, Mundo said, he stopped being involved in other problem behaviors, including drug use.

> A lot of my homies died, got killed. Guns. Actually one of my home boys got shot in the head... and Nick's brother, he was killed. And then the drugs we used to do, like paint, that was a big thing then... once that happened, we all promised we weren't gonna do it, for him.

DISCUSSION AND CONCLUSION

This study illustrates the profound impact of their ethnic identity on the Mexican-American, youth interviewed and on their social interactions. In particular, the data illuminates acculturative stressors including schisms between generations, conflicting expectations in various settings, and issues of conflicting loyalties. Ecologically, these issues emerge on micro, meso, and macro levels, impacting the youth intrapersonally, interpersonally, and in their larger environment. While group solidarity might buffer the intensity of cultural tensions, the data demonstrates a poignant clash between more and less acculturated youth of Mexican origins. Prejudice and stereotypes exist within and outside these groups as well. While many of the conflicts witnessed in this study are of a socio-emotional nature, others manifest as blatant acts of violence—in family, peer, and personal arenas.

Death was a pervasive presence in the lives of the youth in this study in the form of gang violence, suicides, and accidents. However, these youth created meaning out of their stressors and traumas. Many of them described powerful pride in their ethnicity, strong family values, an undercurrent of spirituality, and beliefs that life's hardships prepare one for adulthood. As described throughout this article, resilience abounds in this group.

The first implication of this study for clinicians and researchers is the value of a strengths perspective (Saleeby, 1999). Since much of the literature on Latino/Latina youth comes from a deficit perspective, it is important—despite the clear repercussions of contextual challenges—that resilience be a lens for connecting and intervening with Mexican-American youth. The risk-and-resilience model gives the opportunity for helping-professionals and researchers to shift their focus from concentrating on psychopathology, to an understanding of the process of healthy human development despite environmental challenges (Masten, 1994).

Clearly, more research is needed in the areas of acculturation and acculturative stress and the relationship between these factors and Latino/Latina adolescent development and functioning. The conflicts among adolescents with different acculturative types should be taken into consideration, and orthogonal models (Cuellar and Arnold, 1995; Oetting and Beauvais, 1991) should be considered so as not to oversimplify the picture.

Perhaps the most important implication of this study is that mere awareness of ethnic differences is not enough to intervene effectively with Mexican-American youth. While cultural sensitivity enhances prevention efforts and ethnic matching often maximizes program impact (Botvin, Baker, & Dusenbury, 1995; Botvin, Schinke, & Orland, 1995), how one obtains a clear picture of a culture is critical. It is recommended that naturalistic research be coupled with quantitative research in order to learn the nuances of a particular target group. Latino/Latina youth, when given a chance to have their voices amplified, have powerful insights into their world, their relationships, families, peers, and selves.

REFERENCES

Aguirre, A. & Baker, D. V. (2000). *Structured inequality in the United States: critical discussions and the continuing significance of race, ethnicity, and gender.* Upple Saddle River, New Jersey: Prentice Hall.

Allison, K. R., Adlaf, E. M., and Tates, D. (1997). Life strain, coping, and substance use among high school students. *Addiction Research, 5*(3), 251–272.

Alva, S. A. (1995). Psychological distress and alcohol use in Hispanic adolescents, *Journal of Youth and Adolescents, 24*(4), 481–497.

Avison, W. R. and McAlpine, D. D. (1992). Gender differences in symptoms of depression among adolescents. *Journal of Health and Social behavior, 33*, 77–96.

Barrera, M., Jr. and Reese, F. (1993). Natural social support systems and Hispanic substance abuse. In R. S. Myers, B. L. Kail, & T. D. Watts (Eds.), *Hispanic substance abuse* (pp. 115–130). Springfield, IL: Charles C. Thomas.

Barrera, M., Jr., Li, S. A., and Chassin, L. (1993). Ethnic group differences in vulnerability to parental alcoholism and life stress: A study of hispanic and non-hispanic caucasian adolescents. *American Journal of Community Psychology, 21*, 15–35.

Barrera, M., Jr., Li, S. A., and Chassin, L. (1995). Effects of parental alcoholism and life stress on Hispanic and non-Hispanic Caucasian adolescents: A prospective study. *American Journal of Community Psychology, 23*, 479–507.

Berardo, F. M. (1991). Family research in the 1980's: Recent trends and future directions. In A. Booth (Ed.), *Contemporary families: Looking forward, looking back.* Minneapolis: National Council on Family Relations.

Berry, J.W. (1980). Acculturation as Varieties of Adaptation. In A.M. Padilla (Ed.), *Acculturation: Theory, Models and Some New Findings* (pp. 9–25). Boulder, CO: Westview.

Berry, J. and Kim, U. (1988). Acculturation and mental health. In P. Dasen, J. W. Bery, & N. Sartorius (Eds.), *Cross-cultural psychology and health: Towards applications* (pp. 207–236). London: Sage.

Botvin, G. J., Baker, E., and Dusenbury, L. (1995). Long-term follow up results of a randomized drug abuse prevention trial in a white middle class population. *Journal of the American Medical Association, 273*(14), 1106–1112.

Botvin, G. J., Schinke, S., and Orlandi, M. A. (1995). *Drug abuse prevention with multiethnic youth.* Sage: Thousand Oaks, London, New Dehli.

Bry, B. H., McKeon, P., and Pandina, R. J. (1982). Extent of drug use as a function of number of risk factors. *Journal of Abnormal Psychology, 91*, 273–279.

Burnam, M. A., Hough, R. L., Karno, M., Escobar, J. I., and Teller, C. H. (1987). Acculturation and the lifetime prevalence of psychiatric disorders among Mexican Americans in Los Angeles. *Journal of Health and Social Behavior, 28*, 89–102.

Carvajal, S. C., Hanson, C. E., Romero, A. J., and Coyle, K. K. (2002). Behavioural risk factors and protective factors in adolescents: A comparison of Latinos and non-Latino Whites. *Ethnicity & Health, 7*(3), 181–193.

Centers for Disease Control and Prevention. (1996). Youth risk behavior surveillance. *Morbidity and Mortality Weekly Report*: United States 1995, *45*, 1–84.

Cowen, E. L. and Work, W. (1988). Resilient children, psychological wellness, and primary preventions. *American Journal of Community Psychology, 16*, 591–607.

Cuellar, I. and Arnold, B. (1995). Acculturation Rating Scale for Mexican Americans-II: A revision of the original ARSMA scale. *Hispanic Journal of Behavioral Sciences, 17*(3), 275–305.

D'Arcy, C. and Siddique, C. M. (1984). Psychological distress among Canadian adolescents. *Psychological Medicine, 14*, 615–628.

Denzin, N. K. and Lincoln, Y. S (Eds.) (1994). *Handbook of qualitative research.* Thousand Oaks, London, New Delhi: Sage Publications.

Falicov, C. J. (1996). Mexican families. In M. McGoldrick, J. Giordano, & J. K. Pearce (Eds.), *Ethnicity and family therapy* (2nd ed.). New York: The Guilford Press.

Feliz-Ortiz, M. and Newcomb, M. D. (1992). Risk and protective factors in drug use among Latino and white adolescents. *Hispanic Journal of Behavioral Science, 14*, 291–309.

Freire, P. (1993). Pedagogy of the oppressed. New York: Continuum.

Galguera, T. (1998). Students' attitudes toward teachers' ethnicity, bilinguality, and gender. *Hispanic Journal of Behavioral Sciences, 20*, 411–428.

Gilbert, J. M. and Cervantes, R. C. (1986). Patterns and practices of alcohol use among Mexican Americans: A comprehensive review. *Hispanic Journal of Behavioral Sciences, 8,* 1–60.

Glaser, B. and Strauss, A. (1967). *The discovery of grounded theory.* Chicago, Illinois: Aldine. Denzin, N. K. and Lincoln, Y. S. (Eds.) (1994). *Hand book of qualitative research.* Thousand Oaks, London, New Delhi: Sage Publications.

Greene, R. R. and Conrad, A. P. (2001). Basic assumptions and terms. In R. R. Greene (Ed.), *Resiliency: An integrated approach to practice, policy, and research* (pp. 29–62). Washington, DC: NASW Press.

Hawkins, J. D., Catalano, R. F., and Miller, J. Y. (1992). Risk and protective factors for alcohol and other drug problems in adolescence and early adulthood: Implications for substance abuse prevention. *Psychological Bulletin, 112*(1), 64–105.

Holleran, L. K., Kim, Y., and Dixon, K. (2004). Innovative approaches to risk assessment within alcohol prevention programming. In A. R. Roberts & K. R. Yeager (Eds.), *Evidence-based practice manual: Research and outcome measures in health and human services.* New York: Oxford University Press.

Holleran, L. and Waller, M. A. (2003). Sources of resilience of Chicano/a youth: Forging identities in the borderlands. *Child and Adolescent Social Work Journal, 20*(5), 335–350.

Horowitz, R. (1983). *Honor and the American dream: Culture and identity in a Chicano community.* New Brunswick, NJ: Rutgers University Press.

Hunt, G., Joe, K., and Waldorf, D. (1996). "Drinking, kicking back, and gang banging: alcohol, violence, and street gangs. *Free Inquiry in Creative Sociology, 24*(2), 123–132.

Jessor, R. (1993). Successful adolescent development among youth in high-risk settings. *American Psychologist, 48*(2), 117–126.

Kercher, G. A. and McShane, M. (1984). The prevalence of child sexual abuse victimization in an adult sample of Texas residents. *Child Abuse and Neglect, 8,* 495–501.

Lofland, J. and Lofland, L. (1995). *Analyzing social settings: A guide to qualitative observation and analysis.* Belmont, CA: Wadsworth, Inc.

Lorion, R. P., Price, R. H., and Eaton, W. W. (1989). The prevention of child and adolescent disorders: From theory to research. In D. Shaffer, I. Philips, & N. B. Enzer (Eds.), *Prevention of mental disorders, alcohol and other drug use in children and adolescents* (pp. 55–59). Rockville, MD: Office of Substance Abuse Prevention and American Academy of Child and Adolescent Psychiatry, Prevention Monograph #2 (DHHS Publication No. ADM89–1646).

Marsiglia, F. F., Kulis, S., and Hecht, M. L. (2001). Ethnic labels and ethnic identity as predictors of drug use among middle school students in the Southwest. *Journal of Research on Adolescence, 11*(1), 21–48.

Masten, A. S. (1994). Resilience in individual development: Successful adaptation despite risk and adversity. In M. C. Wang & E. W. Gorden (Eds.), *Educational resilience in inner-city America: Challenge and prospects, 1994.* Hillsdale, NJ: Erlbaum.

Mirandé, A. (1985). *The Chicano experience: An alternative perspective.* Norte Dame, N: University of Notre Dame Press.

Oetting, E.R. and Beauvais, F. (1991). Orthogonal cultural identification theory: The cultural Acculturation Status on Delinquency for Mexican-American Adolescents. *American Journal of Community Psychology, 27*(2), 189–211.

Ortiz, V. and Arce, C. H. (1984). Language orientation and mental health status among persons of Mexican descent. *Hispanic Journal of Behavioral Sciences, 6*(2), 127–143.

Olmos, E. J., Ybarra, L., and Monterrey, M. (1999). *Americanos: Latino life in the United States.* Boston, MA: Little, Brown.

Perez, D. M. (2001). Ethnic differences in property, violent, and sex offending for abused and nonabused adolescents. *Journal of Criminal Justice, 29,* 407–417.

Phinney, J. (1996). When we talk about American ethnic groups what do we mean? *American Psychologist, 51,* 918–927.

Redfield, R., Linton, R., and Herskovits, M. J. (1936). Memorandum for the study of acculturation. *American Anthropologist, 38,* 149–152.

Rodriguez, D. (2000). Searching for sanctuaries: Cruising through town in a red convertible. Sandoval-Sanctez, A. and Sternbach, N. S. (Eds.) *Puro teatro: a latina anthology,* 313–318. Tuscon, Arizona: The University of Arizona Press.

Rogler, L. H., Cortes, D., and Malgady, R. G. (1991). Acculturation and mental health status among Hispanics. *American Psychologist, 46*(6), 585–597.

Romanucci-Ross, L. and DeVos, G. (Eds.) (1995). *Ethnic identity: Creation, conflict and accommodation.* Walnut Creek, London, New Delhi: Altamira Press.

Saleebey, D. (1997). *The strengths perspective in social work practice.* New York: Longman.

Stavans, I. (1995). *The Hispanic condition: Reflections on culture & Identity in America.* New York: Harper Perrenial.

Strauss, A.L. (1987). *Qualitative analysis for social scientists.* Cambridge: Cambridge University Press.

Suárez-Orozco, M. (1989). Towards a psychosocial understanding of Hispanic adaptation to American schooling. In H. T. Trueba (Ed.), *Success or failure? Learning and the language minority student* (pp. 156–168). Cambridge, MA: Newbury House.

Suárez-Orozco, C. and Suárez-Orozco, M. (1995). *Transformations: Immigration, family life and achievement motivation and achievement.* Stanford: Stanford University Press.

Taylor, V. L., Hurley, E. C., and Riley, M. T. (1986). The influence of acculturation upon the adjustment of preschool Mexican American children of single-parent families. *Family Therapy, 13,* 249–256.

Vélez-Ibáñez, C. G. (1996). *Border visions: Mexican cultures of the Southwest United States.* Tucson, AZ.: The University of Arizona Press.

Vega, W. A., Zimmerman, R., Warheit, G., and Gil, A. (1995, August 17–19). *Acculturation, stress and Latino adolescent drug use.* Paper presented at the Social Stressors, personal and Social Resources and their Health consequences, Bethesda, MD.

Vidich, A. J. and Lyman, S. M. (1994). Qualitative methods: Their history in sociology and anthropology. In Denzin, N. K. & Lincoln, Y. S (Eds.), *Handbook of qualitative research* (p. 23–59). Thousand Oaks, London, New Delhi: Sage Publications.

Waller, M. (2001). Resilience in ecosystemic context: Evolution of the concept. *American Journal of Orthopsychiatry, 71*(3), 1–8.

Warheit, G., Vega, W., Auth, J., and Meinhardt, K. (1985). Mexican-American immigration and mental health: A comparative analysis of psychosocial stress and dysfunction. In W. Vega & M. Miranda (Eds.), *Stress and Hispanic mental health*. Rockville, MD: National Institute of mental Health.

Wong, S. K. (1999). Acculturation rating scale for Mexican Americans - II: A revision of the original ARSMA scale. *Journal of Behavioral Sciences, 17*(3), 275–304.

4

The Prevalence of HIV Among Substance-Abusing African-American Women: A Qualitative Investigation

JENNY L. JONES

University of Tennessee, College of Social Work, 193E Polk Ave., Nashville

African-American women represent the fastest growing segment of the population of individuals who are infected with HIV in the United States. This increased rate of infection can largely be attributed to risk behaviors related to substance use and heterosexual contact with male partners who are injection drug users. The literature documents that substance abuse has a strong link to HIV/AIDS in the United States (CDC, 2004; Jones, 2004; McNair & Prather, 2004). The ongoing use and misuse of alcohol and other drugs often reduces one's decision-making abilities and increases sexual risk-taking that can ultimately lead to an HIV/AIDS diagnosis (Avins et al., 1997; Jermott & Brown, 2003). In 2001, 42,983 new cases of AIDS was reported to the Centers for Disease Control and Prevention (CDC), nearly one-fifth (17.4%) of which were among injection drug users (IDUs; CDC, 2001a). Divided by gender, 31,901 new AIDS cases were reported for men, and IDU's accounted for approximately 20% of these new cases. Of the total number of new cases reported for women IDU's accounted for 11,082 (20%).

During the past decade, HIV infection among women in the United States has significantly increased, especially among communities of color. Of the 42,983 new cases reported in 2001, 69.1% were among people of color (African Americans, Hispanics, Asian/Pacific Islanders, and American Indians/Alaskan Natives; CDC, 2001b). Disaggregating data by gender, indi-cates that African Americans are by far the most affected group, with African-American women representing over 60% of new cases and African-American men representing approximately 44% of new cases reported, respectively, for men and women. The injection drug-use exposure category, reflect that African-American women made up almost 57% of all new AIDS cases for women, and African-American men made up 52% of all new AIDS cases for men.

The rates of new HIV cases for people of color appear to be very similar to those of the new cases of AIDS. Here again, African-American women appear to be the most impacted. In 2001, African-American women repre-sented 64% of the 11,133 new HIV infection cases (CDC, 2001b). Overall, the rates of HIV and AIDS cases have been overwhelmingly higher among African Americans than among any other racial and ethnic group in the United States (CDC, 1987; Estrada, 2002; Jones, 2004), and African American-women, more so than all other women, particularly appear to be most vulnerable to HIV infection.

HIV/AIDS is categorized in the literature as a severe life threatening illness (Carbone, 2001), and can potentially be viewed as a chronic state of stress, with substance abuse and traumatic experiences being among the risk factors for African-American women. For many African-American women, early life trauma plays a critical role in how and when they fall victim to the ravages of substance abuse. Violent physical abuse and sexual abuse afflict large numbers of African American women, who at any age are at a much greater risk than other groups of women for rape and sexual abuse; are three times more likely to report a rape (Davis, 1997), and according to FBI records are more likely than any other group of women to be raped. Because of these traumatic experiences, compounded with substance abuse, African-American women experience HIV in a chronic state of stress.

Risk factors for HIV/AIDS are exacerbated among women of color. Historically women of color have been adversely affected by disenfranchise-ment, marginalization, and poverty. These issues have played a significant role in the tendency for the health concerns of women of color to be unrecognized or under-represented in health care planning. Often, the care provided has not been consistent. This practice, in turn, has caused a domino effect of neglect and institutionalized prejudice against women and people of color. One result is the creation of an invisible, yet continuously growing, population of women of color who face high HIV morbidity and mortality rates.

The current epidemiology trends of the HIV/AIDS epidemic as it relates to women, more specifically African American women in the United States has reached alarming rates. Injection drug use, most notably is the second leading exposure category for HIV/AIDS among African American women (CDC, 2002). Researchers have identified several factors that influence African American womens' heightened risk of acquiring HIV/AIDS (Land, 2000; McNair & Prather, 2004; Pequegnat & Stover, 1999). These factors are related to the conjunction of gender, race, and social class in the lives of African-American women, giving rise to conditions within their social environment such as stress, poverty, poor health (Logan et al., 20002), and concurrent drug use and mental health issues (U.S. Department of Health Human Services, 2004). Recent epidemiological studies have shown that between 30 and 60 percent of drug users have concurrent mental health diagnoses, including personality disorders, major depression, schizophrenia and bi-polar disorder (Leshner, 2000). In women, these factors may be exacerbated due to the multiple demands associated with child rearing and caregiving, which frequently result in stress and role strain that test the physical and emotional capabilities of women. Pejorative attitudes, practices, and discrimination are intensified toward women because it is assumed that most HIV-affected women are also members of other stigmatized groups, namely, injecting drug users or sexual partners of IDUs, women of color, poor women, sexual partners of bisexual men, and women who previously led a lifestyle of sexual indiscretion (Campbell, 1999; Jones, 2002).

The influential role of the factors stated above, as they relate to illicit drug use, has well been documented, highlighting the vulnerability faced by African-American women residing in communities characterized by high levels of poverty, crime, and violence (Brown et al., 1999; Jones, (in press); Pequegnat & Schpoznick, 2000), along with poor access to services (health and social; Land, 2000), and resources (housing and education; Minar, 2002).

Another contextual factor that has had an impact on the experience of African American women in social environments is their relationships with significant others. This is the framework for the emergence of contextual factors that influence risky behavior. In some instances, contextual factors such as victimization history (e.g., experiencing sexual or physical abuse) can affect some individuals similarly, however they are most properly conceptualized as unique features of one's history that influence their perspective (Logan et al., 2002; Roberts, 1999). For example, sexual assault is associated with increased risk-taking among women (Wyatt et al., 2002). The experience of sexual assault can be viewed as an important feature of a woman's history, influencing her behavior and cognition regarding sexual behavior and risk taking. In this way, her history of sexual assault is a contextual factor—one that is of significance for her. These factors are linked to heightened risk for traumatic exposure (Davis, 1997).

For African-American women, a history that includes exposure to trauma is a predictor of the likelihood of becoming infected with HIV (Wyatt et al., 2002). Trauma related to childhood physical experiences, as well sexual abuse and or intimate partner abuse in adulthood, is related to increased risk for HIV infection among women. McNair and Prather (2004), hypothesized that one mechanism for this relationship is women's use of drugs as a means for coping with the emotional consequences of abuse; consequently substance use impairs one's decision making ability, thus leaving women vulnerable to sexual risk taking, which can ultimately lead to HIV infection.

Other environmental factors that are connected with African American women's HIV risk are issues such as poverty and drug use. Based on their review of a study of the relationship between trauma and HIV infection among women living in the South Bronx, Brown, Peterside et al.'s, (2002) indicate the interconnection of environment and risk for these women. Their findings reveal that women identified as high risk and HIV negative also reported high lifetime rates of trauma, as well as HIV risk behaviors such as unprotected sex, multiple sex partners, crack cocaine use, and sex exchange for drugs. Together these risk behaviors appear to initiate from the environmental stresses associated with these women's living conditions.

The epidemiological and social contextual factors highlighted in this paper document the significance that substance abuse and the heightened risks for HIV infection and exposure to trauma play in the lives of African-American women, both infected and affected by HIV/AIDS. This paper reports findings of a qualitative study comprised of HIV infected African American women with self-reported histories of illicit drug use. The women in this study described their HIV status as being a result of their drug use. The findings from this study should be useful to service providers as they strive to design and provide effective interventions to help African American women cope with the special challenges posed by substance use and HIV/AIDS infection.

METHOD

Data used in the current analyses were collected as a part of a study aimed at assessing the impact of maternal HIV/AIDS diagnosis on the mental health needs of affected children and families, which included a supplemental qualitative analysis on HIV disclosure and coping. The study included HIV positive women who received care services. (i.e., health care and case management from various AIDS Service Organizations (ASOs) throughout metro Atlanta, Georgia). To be eligible for inclusion in the study, the women must have identified as HIV infected and have a child living with them between the ages of 4–18. This paper includes baseline data collected from the 28 women who were interviewed between January and March 2002.

Data Collection

Semi-structured interviews were held with 28 African American women that were primary caregivers for children ages 4–18 years. The women were recruited from various health clinics in the metro Atlanta area that provide care for HIV infected persons. The women were solicited for the study via flyers being placed in the waiting areas of the clinic, and case managers also distributed flyers during clinic appointments. The flyers listed a contact number instructing the women to contact the researcher directly if they were interested in participating in the study. Once contact was established, the purpose of the study was discussed along with issues of confidentiality and consent for participation. The study participants were assured that participation in the study was on a voluntary basis and their identity and responses would be kept confidential. The women were also informed that neither agreement nor refusal to participate in the study would affect services received from any of the programs in which they were enrolled. The participants were given an incentive (5 bus tokens) for participation in the study. If a woman agreed to participate in the study, an appointment was made to meet at a location agreed upon by she and the researcher. After obtaining written informed consent, the interview process began using a semi-structured interview guide.

Development of the key informant interview questions was guided by the research reviewed earlier on maternal HIV diagnosis and its impact on the mental health needs of affected children and family members, and the impact of disclosure and coping.

Demographic information was gathered through a two-page pencil and paper survey containing 18 items developed by the author expressly for the purpose of this study. Items on the survey asked standard demographic information regarding the respondents' age, ethnicity, personal household income, religious affiliation, and highest-grade level earned. The survey also gathered information about the respondent's HIV status and age of children.

MEASURES

To gain a better understanding of the women and the contextual factors that impact their lives, seven marker variables were used: ethnicity, age, educational level, number of years the women had been infected, number of symptoms reported by the women is used as a health and psychological marker, (i.e., describe the number of symptoms exhibited in the last six months), whether the woman had received an AIDS (not HIV) diagnosis, and the number of years of having an AIDS diagnosis.

Detailed information was obtained about the mother's decision to disclose her HIV status to their children and family. And, if the woman had not disclosed her status information was gathered to reflect the reasons she had not. The interview also focused on questions pertaining to coping strategies among the children and family members who had been told the diagnosis. Data was also collected about the experience the women had had since being diagnosed with HIV. Raw data from the interviews included tape recordings and field notes, which were transcribed verbatim. After transcribing the tapes a thorough reading, with several re-reads and annotation of codable topics, themes, and issues was conducted. The qualitative responses were coded using grounded theory methods (Glaser & Straus, 1997). These data were analyzed for content: a list of codes was first created for each open-ended question; the codes were then categorized to reflect key themes. This process involved a systematic classification of things, persons, events, and important characteristics of these items seeking similar and dissimilar patterns. The mechanism used to facilitate the process of systematic classification is standard procedure when analyzing qualitative data (Berg, 2001; Padgett, 1998). To maximize data reliability the researcher set up several sheets of papers separately, with major topics of interest and several other sub-topics or themes. Consistent with qualitative research, the researcher had no specific hypotheses developed beforehand. The analysis consisted of a comparative method between two independent raters. Each rater separately identified patterns, consistencies, and inconsistencies that served as a basis for identifiable themes. Then a comparative method among raters was performed to determine which relations were consistently observed.

RESULTS

Descriptive Analyses

The demographic characteristics of the study sample are reflected below in Table 1. Twenty-eight African-American women from metro Atlanta participated in the current study. Collectively, these women had 51 children. The following information was obtained from key informants: number of children in the family; socioeconomic status; religious affiliation; and type of family with respect to number and status of parents infected with AIDS.

INFORMANT CHARACTERISTICS

Of the twenty-eight participants, 18% ($n = 5$) were grandmothers and 82% ($n = 23$) were mothers. Ages of the informants ranged from 26 to 58, with a mean of 37.11 and standard deviation of 7.55. The mode was 32. The ethnic breakdown was 100% ($n = 28$) African-American women (see Table 1). The number of years reported by the respondent with an HIV diagnosis ranged from 2 months to 19 years with a mean of 6.94 and a standard deviation of 4.367.

Table 1 provides information regarding the educational level of the women. Sixty-one percent ($n = 17$) graduated form high school, 21% ($n = 6$) had some college training and 11% ($n = 3$) had other training (i.e., vocational education).

Table 2 describes the number of symptoms displayed by the infected women in the six months prior to the time during which the study was conducted. Fifty-seven percent ($n = 16$) displayed no symptoms, whereas 36% ($n = 10$) displayed 1–3 symptoms and 7% ($n = 2$) displayed 4–6

TABLE 1 Demographics of Participants ($N = 28$)

Variable	N	%
Age		
18–30	6	21.0
31–43	17	61.0
44–58	5	18.0
Gender		
Female	28	100.0
Marital status		
Never married	17	61.0
Married (common law married)	1	4.0
Divorced	6	21.0
Separated	2	7.0
Widowed	2	7.0
Children		
Yes	28	100.0
No	0	0.0
Age of children		
Pre-school (4–5)	3	6.0
Child (6–11)	26	51.0
Adolescent (12–18)	22	43.0
Income		
0 to 7,999	17	60.7
8,000 to 16,000	10	35.7
17,000 to 24,000	1	3.6
Mother's education level		
Elementary	1	4.0
High School	17	61.0
Some College	6	21.0
Post Graduate	1	4.0
Other	3	10.0
Religious affiliation		
Baptist	15	54.0
Christian	6	21.0
Catholic	2	7.0
Other	3	11.0
No religious affiliation	2	7.0

TABLE 2 Number of Symptoms Exhibited in the Last Six Months by Infected Person

Category	N	%
No symptoms	16	57
1–3 symptoms	10	36
4–6 symptoms	2	7
Total	28	100

symptoms. Generally, people infected with HIV will be visibly ill when displaying four to six symptoms. This decrease in the number of symptoms was partly due to the new medications prescribed over the past 5–7 years.

With respect to the AIDS diagnosis, 39% ($n = 11$) of the 28 infected women had received their medical status from their doctor. The number of years for those diagnosed with AIDS ranged from 2 months to 12 years with a mean of 2.28 years and standard deviation of 1.24297. The remaining 61% ($n = 17$) were currently diagnosed with HIV.

Throughout the interviews several themes emerged from the conversations that the women reported about disclosure, however the issue of substance abuse emerged as a compelling sub-theme related to most of the responses. A substance abuse history was self-disclosed by 70% (20) of the women. All of them attributed their HIV diagnosis to their past drug use.

SUBSTANCE USE: THE PRECURSOR

The interaction of substance abuse, HIV infection, and trauma requires further exploration. For many African American women, early life trauma plays a critical role in how and why they fall victim to the devastation of substance abuse. Several of the women in this study-discussed their feelings about prior substance abuse history and how this was connected to receiving an HIV diagnosis as: "I had been using since I was 18 and I knew it was just a matter of time," stated Mary, a 45-year-old grandmother who cares for her two grandchildren. Eileen, another 48-year-old grandmother, who provides care for her two grandchildren stated, "I've done drugs. I shot up drugs for thirty, close to thirty-five years, so being infected with this is just a part of it, you know, to be honest." Both of these women reported they began using drugs at an early age as a result of poor relationships with their mothers and the men in their mother's lives. Mary stated, "my mother's old man use to get drunk and mess with me and my lil' sister. When I got old enough I got out of there and took my sister with me. I started using right after I got out there; it was the only way I could deal with it. I couldn't believe my mother would sit back let him do that." When you are out on the streets you have to fend for yourself couple of the women shared experiences about the child welfare agency that had removed their children due to their repeated drug use. Kathy stated, "When I was in my addiction I lost my children to the system. My mother had to take custody of them. They used to see me out on the streets high, begging for drugs. I put my kids through a lot. When I first found out I had this virus, I didn't stop using. It took me a while. But, I finally got it together and got myself clean, got my children back, and got a second chance at life."

Another theme that emerged related to the ongoing use of illicit drugs and HIV/AIDS was that many of the women's families had suffered the loss of a loved one from HIV/AIDS, therefore the women were quite conscious of HIV/AIDS. One woman, Tanya, explained that her family members (mother and aunt) still have a difficult time saying the words HIV, inspite of the fact that "my cousin Jimmy died in January, two years ago of AIDS. He had shot drugs for a long time. Since he has been dead, my family will talk about his death, but rarely do they say the word HIV, rather they say Jimmy used those drugs until he killed himself. The fact that he used drugs appeared to be much more accepting for my aunt than he died of AIDS."

A number of the women spoke about the relationships they had with their mothers, which were often times very complex. These feelings are further exacerbated when illicit drug use is involved. Anita, a 33-year old mother of three stated, "when I first told my mother that I had HIV she said, 'I knew something like this would probably happen one day if I continued to stay out there and use drugs.' She was right, because that's how I contracted the virus." Bertha, a 29-year old mother of one explained, "people treat you different when you have HIV"; "they think they can catch it from you by shaking your hand. My mother served me food in paper plates, or she would wash my cup immediately after I used it. This made me feel bad. However, when I was in my addiction I didn't think much about it.' I didn't go around my family much when I was out there."

DISCUSSION

Several themes emerged from the analyses that have relevance to a feminist perspective, meaning that the women spoke openly about issues that had importance for them. Most importantly, HIV/AIDS is a salient issue for substance abusing women interviewed in this sample. The women in this study spoke extensively about their substance abuse histories and how they believed this contributed to their HIV diagnosis. These women's construction of the process of substance abuse and its influence on their behavior in some ways is viewed as a natural part of their lives.

The abuse of illicit substances, for many of them is a self-medicating strategy to dull painful feelings resulting from exposure to a traumatic event. The exposure to such events is directly related to the connection of gender, race, and social class in the lives of African-American women, giving rise to conditions within their social environment such as stress, poverty, poor health and concurrent drug use and mental health issues. These factors have been noted by a number of researchers (Brown, Peterside et al., 2002; Logan et al., 2002; McNair & Prather, 2004; Roberts, 1999; Wyatt et al., 2002). An effective women's health agenda is needed to reverse the adverse and often time complicated systems (i.e., health care, child welfare, drug treatment, etc.) these women must face while seeking help.

Overall, these findings suggest that the interaction of HIV diagnosis and substance abuse is a painful reality for many of the women in this study. Furthermore, African Americans in general are at great risk for traumatic exposure, because of their urban dwelling. For women with HIV infection, it is critical that this factor be taken into consideration, as the literature documents that most HIV-infected women reside in poor inner-city neighborhoods plagued with crime, prostitution, and illicit drug use and sales. These findings further suggest that drug users, particularly women who are HIV-infected are at increased risk for traumatic exposure due to the acquisition of the drugs (illegal drug market), and consumption of drugs (vulnerability and propensity for drugs). This holds especially true for the women in this study, in that many of them described the risk to which they put themselves and their children while using illegal substances.

The painful past experiences of African-American women may have led to subsequent substance abuse problems for these women. Nevertheless, issues related to substance abuse problems among women continue not to be holistically addressed. As noted, HIV is of particular concern for African-American women who abuse substances, however, most efforts regarding HIV are directed toward prevention. This includes condom use, abstinence, and avoidance of body fluids. For women engaged in behavior predicated on lack of self worth and self-esteem, these efforts are too little and too late.

IMPLICATION FOR PRACTICE

African-American women represent disproportionate numbers of women with HIV infection and AIDS. Several factors related to economics, poor health, access to healthcare, and other social and environmental factors impact the lives of African-American women and increase their risk for contracting HIV. Because of these factors, the development and implementation of appropriate strategies to address these issues may be a great challenge for practitioners. Efforts to reach women who are substance users and at risk for HIV must be culturally responsive and they must include approaches that will address the social and environmental factors affecting these women's lives. Doing so will have positive psychological, physical, and social effects that can resonate in the lives of African-American women, their children and families, and their communities.

ACKNOWLEDGEMENTS

The author wishes to acknowledge the assistance of her dissertation chair, Dr. Richard Lyle (Clark Atlanta University) and committee members: Dr. Sarita Davis (Clark Atlanta University) and Dr. Eleen Yancey (Morehouse School of Medicine). This research could not have been completed without the assistance of the multiple AIDS Service Organizations (ASOs) in Metro Atlanta, Georgia.

REFERENCES

Avins, A. L., Lindan, C. P., Woods, W. J., Hudes, E. S., Boscarino, J. A., and Kay, J., et al. (1997). Changes in HIV-related behaviors among heterosexual alcoholics following addiction treatment. *Drug Alcohol Dependence, 44*(1), 47–55.

Berg, B. L. (2001). *Qualitative research methods for the social sciences* (4th ed.). Boston: Allyn and Bacon.

Brown-Peterside, P., Ren, L., Chiasson, M. A., and Koblin, B. (2002). Double Trouble: Violent and non-violent traumas among women at sexual risk of HIV infection. *Women & Health, 36*, 51–64.

Campbell, C. A. (1999). *Women, families, and HIV/AIDS: A sociological perspective on the epidemic in America.* Cambridge, UK: Cambridge University Press.

Carbone, D. (2001). Aftershock: The long-term reactions to traumatic events. *In the body: An AIDS and HIV information resource, 14*(11), 1–64. Retrieved from http://www.thebody.com/bp/nov01/aftershoch.html

Centers for Disease Control and Prevention (CDC). (1987, December 18). *Morbidity and Mortality Weekly Report, 36*(6), 1–20. Atlanta, GA.

Centers for Disease Control and Prevention (CDC). (2001a). *HIV/AIDS among U.S. women: Minority and young women at continuing risk, Year-end 2000.* Atlanta, GA.

Centers for Disease Control and Prevention (CDC). (2001b). *HIV/AIDS surveillance report.* Atlanta, GA.

Centers for Disease Control and Prevention (CDC). (2002). *HIV/AIDS Report.* Atlanta, GA: CSC. Retrieved April 5, 2004, from http://www.cdc.gpv/hiv/stats/hasrsupp51/charts.htm

Centers for Disease Control and Prevention (CDC). (2003). *Basic statistics-exposure categories.* http://www.cdc.gov/hiv/stats/exposure.htm

Davis, R. E. (1997). Trauma and addiction experiences of African American women. *Western Journal of Nursing Research, 19*(4), 442–460.

Estrada, A. L. (2002). Epidemiology of HIV/AIDS, hepatitis B, hepatitis C, and tuberculosis among minority injection drug users. *Public Health Reports, 117*(Suppl. 1), S126–S134.

Glaser, B. G. and Straus, A. L. (1997). *The discovery of grounded theory: Strategies for qualitative research.* Chicago: Aldine.

Jermmott, L. S. and Brown, E. J. (2003). Reducing HIV sexual risk among African American women who use drugs: Hearing their voices. *Journal of the Association of Nurses in AIDS Care, 14*(1), 19–26.

Jones, D. J. (2004). HIV Risk-Reduction Strategies for Substance Abusers: Effecting Behavior Change. *Journal of Black Psychology, 30*(1), 59–77.

Jones, J. L. (2002). *A Study of mental health factors in healthy African American Children and adolescents affected by maternal HIV/AIDS diagnosis.* Unpublished doctoral dissertation.

Jones, J. L. (in press). HIV/AIDS and Women' Health. In C. S. Carter (Ed.), *Social Work and Women's Health* (pp. 88–116). Washington, DC: NASW Press.

Land, H. (2000). AIDS and women of color. In V. J. Lynch (Ed.), *HIV/AIDS at year 2000: A sourcebook for social workers* (pp. 79–96). Boston: Allyn and Bacon.

Leshner, A. (2000). Drug abuse and mental health disorders: comorbidity is reality. NIDA Notes, 14(4). Retrieved from www.drugabuse.gov/NIDA_Notes/NNVol14N4/DirRepVol14N.html

McNair, L. D. and Prather, C. M. (2004). African American Women and AIDS: Factors Influencing Risk and Reaction to HIV Disease. *Journal of Black Psychology, 30*(1), 106–123.

Padgett, D. K. (1998). *Qualitative methods in social work research: Challenges and rewards.* Thousand Oaks, CA: Sage.

Pequegnat, W. and Stover, E. (1999). Considering women's contextual and cultural issues in HIV/STD prevention research. *Cultural Diversity and Ethnic Minority Psychology, 5*, 287–291.

Pequegnant, W. and Szapocznik, J. (2000). The role of families in preventing and adapting to HIV/AIDS: Issues and answers. In W. Pequegnat & J. Szapocznick (Eds.), *Working with families in the era of HIV/AIDS* (pp. 3–26). Thousand Oaks: Sage.

Roberts, C. A. (1999). Drug use among inner-city African American women: The process of managing loss. *Qualitative Health Research, 9*(5), 620–638.

U.S. Department of Health and Human Services. (2004). *Substance Abuse and HIV/AIDS.* Retrieved April 12, 3004, from http://www.hab.hrsa.gov/programs/factsheets/substancefact.htm

Wyatt, G. E., William, J. K., Loeb, T., Carmona, J., Chin, D., and Presley, N., et al. (2002). Does history of trauma contribute to HIV risk for women of color? Implications for prevention and policy. *American Journal of Public Health, 92*, 660–665.

5

Factors Associated with Trauma Symptoms Among Runaway/Homeless Adolescents

SANNA J. THOMPSON

University of Texas at Austin School of Social Work, Austin, Texas, USA

Runaway/homeless adolescents are some of this nation's most vulnerable youth. Prevalence rates are difficult to determine as the definition of 'runaway' and 'homeless' varies (Lifson & Halcón, 2001); however, one national survey found that 7.6% of adolescents 12–17 years of age had spent at least one night in an emergency shelter, public place, abandoned building, or with a stranger during the previous year (Ringwalt, Greene, Robertson, & McPheeters, 1998). Estimates indicate that there are between 500,000 to two million runaway/homeless youth at any time in the U.S. (Farrow, Deisher, Brown, Kulig, & Kipke, 1992). Regardless of the exact number of these youth, they are a group of youth living in precarious and often abusive situations.

Runaway/homeless youth often suffer from exposure to chronic family distress and confront numerous traumatic events in their lives (Williams, Lindsey, Kurtz, & Jarvis, 2001). These youth often characterize their homes as exhibiting interfamily conflict, poor communication, dysfunction, abuse and/or neglect (Rotheram-Borus, 1993; Whitbeck, Hoyt, & Ackley, 1997). For some of these young people, leaving is not a choice. They are pushed out of their homes by parents encouraging them to leave, abandoning them, or subjecting them to intolerable levels of mistreatment (Dadds, Braddock, Cuers, Elliott, & Kelly, 1993; Rotheram-Borus, 1993). The struggles within these families often reflect a high degree of family discord and lack of emotional cohesion and warmth (Crespi & Sabatelli, 1993; Dadds et al., 1993; Janus, Archambault, Brown, & Welsh, 1995; Whitbeck et al., 1997). For some adolescents the dangers of the streets are more attractive than remaining in an environment characterized by parental dysfunction and maltreatment (Whitbeck & Simons, 1990).

Runaway/homeless youth experience destructive forces that impede their growth and development, such as delinquency, risky sexual experiences, victimization, and violence (Whitbeck & Hoyt, 1999). Running away creates its own stressors. Even leaving a chaotic family is tremendously disruptive as it creates the loss of familiar routines of school attendance, family life, and daily contact with friends. These youth often develop a heightened sense of vulnerability, anxiety, anger, and fear (Whitbeck & Hoyt, 2000) and experience elevated rates of distress, delinquency, and substance use (MacLean, Paradise, & Cauce, 1999). Anxiety reactions, aggression, withdrawal, dissociative reactions, and depression are common among youth living in stressful situations (Richters, 1993) and are similar to those of children with histories of maltreatment and physical/sexual abuse (Downey & Walker, 1992). Exposure to these types of traumatic events or victimization may produce symptoms of acute stress or post traumatic stress disorder (PTSD; Green, 1993; Mundy, Robertson, Robertson, & Greenblatt, 1990).

Posttraumatic stress is typically manifested by symptoms of intrusive thoughts and persistent re-experiencing of traumatic events, nightmares, hyper vigilance, and attempting to avoid negative thoughts or memories (American Psychiatric Association, 1994). Research has suggested an association between trauma and substance use (Kilpatrick et al., 2000; Stewart et al., 2004). Adolescents who live outside of familial homes in unstable, even abusive, situations often engage in a variety of high-risk behaviors, including substance use (Greene, Ennett, & Ringwalt, 1999). Illicit drug has been recognized as a negative method of coping with life on the street (Berkman & Kawachi, 2000). Rates of alcohol, marijuana, and other substances use are substantially higher among runaway/homeless youth than their non-runaway peers (Baer, Ginzler, & Peterson, 2003; Greene & Ringwalt, 1997; Johnston, O'Malley, & Bachman, 2002; Ringwalt, Greene, & Robertson, 1998). One study comparing runaway and non-runaway youth found that runaways were three times more likely to use marijuana (43% vs. 15%), seven times more likely to use crack/cocaine (19% vs. 2.6%), five times more likely to use hallucinogens (14% vs. 3.3%), and four times more likely to use heroin (3% vs. 7%) than their non-runaway peers (Forst, 1994). Parents of these youth also use substances, which may have an impact on the young people's use and subsequent consequences as well.

Runaway/homeless youth are at particularly high-risk for developing PTSD symptoms, due to their interfamily conflict or living on the street. In one study, 83% of street youths were physically and/or sexually victimized after leaving home and approximately 18% of these youths met research criteria for PTSD (Stewart et al., 2004). However, limited research has focused on issues concerning PTSD among runaway/homeless adolescents. To address this gap, the following study questions were posed: 1) what is the level of PTSD; 2) what substance use, family, and youth factors are associated with PTSD; and 3) what is the impact of these factors on PTSD among runaway/homeless youth? Understanding the consequences of stress and trauma on this particularly vulnerable population is needed to develop appropriate and sensitive intervention strategies.

METHODS

Sample and Procedures

The data for this study were collected from consecutive entrants to shelters for runaway youths in two comparable mid-sized cities in New York and Texas. These federally-funded shelters are similar to other youth emergency shelters offering services to runaway youths across the U.S. (Greene et al., 1997). They served approximately ten male and ten female adolescents (ages 12 to 18 years) concurrently and provided basic crisis and counseling services.

Within 48 hours of the youth's admission to the shelter, these agencies were required to contact the youth's parent or guardian. Parental consent for the youth's participation in the study was sought during the initial encounter. Only youths who had received parent consent were approached and recruited for participation. Following the youth's assent, they were asked to complete several brief, self-report questionnaires. One hundred fifty-five ($n = 155$) youths admitted to a shelter in western New York state and 195 youths admitted to a shelter in northern Texas participated. Youths were not approached if they were only seeking short-term respite from parental conflict or abuse and were being returned to parental homes or another long-term residential living situation relatively quickly. Only those identified by shelter staff as runaways and admitted for at least 24 hours were recruited for participation.

Measures

Data were collected from two sources: study questionnaires and agency data. Shelter staff collected information on each youth admitted using the Runaway Homeless Youth Management Information System (RHY MIS). RHY MIS is an automated data collection system developed by the Administration for Children and Families (ACF) and its use is required in all federally funded youth shelters nationwide. Shelter staff recorded information during the intake process, during the youth's shelter stay, and at discharge. RHY MIS variables utilized in this study included basic demographics (age, gender, ethnicity, and the youth's past living situation before admission to the shelter, the number of times the youth ran away, the number of days "on the run," and the number of days the youth stayed in the shelter). Youths also identified specific problems they experienced, such as educational challenges and family difficulties, including physical/sexual abuse or neglect. A series of questions queried each area, which were later coded as whether or not the youth reported a problem in that area. For example, questions associated with education included: "have you had poor grades in school?", "have you ever been told you have a learning disability?", "were you ever been expelled from school?", and "were you ever truant from school?"

The adolescents' traumatic distress and related psychological symptoms were measured using the Trauma Symptom Checklist for Children (TSCC; Briere, 1996). The TSCC consists of trauma-responsive items that assess six psychological affects. These subscales include: 1) anxiety ("How often do I feel afraid something bad might happen?"); 2) depression ("How often do I want to hurt myself; How often do I feel lonely?"); 3) anger ("How often do I argue too much?"); 4) prosttraumatic stress ("How often do I have bad dreams or nightmares?"); 5) dissociation ("How often do I go away in my mind and try not to think?"); and 6) sexual concerns ("How often do I think about having sex?"). The 54 items are rated on a 4-point scale (1 = *never* to 5 = *all of the time*). Internal consistency reliability estimates of the six scales are high; alphas ranged from .77 to .89. Raw scores were converted to T-scores for easier interpretation; the mean of the T-score distribution is 50 and one standard deviation is ten (Briere, 1996).

Substance use of youth and parents (as reported by youth) was also evaluated. Youth reported 'ever using' and 'frequency of use in the past month' for a variety of illicit substances, including cigarettes, alcohol, marijuana, LSD, ecstasy, and inhalants. Parental use was also identified as 'ever use' or 'binge use' for the same substances.

Family characteristics were evaluated using the Family Functioning Scale (FFS; Tavitian, Lubiner, Green, Grebstein, & Velicer, 1987). The FFS consists of 40 items that measure five dimensions of family functioning: 1) positive family affect ("People in my family listen when I speak"); 2) rituals ("We pay attention to traditions in my family"); 3) worries ("I worry when I disagree with the opinions of other family members"); 4) conflicts ("People in my family yell at each other"); and 5) communication ("When I have questions about personal relationships, I talk with my family member"). Respondents rated items on a seven-point scale (1 = *never* to 7 = *always*) and items were summed for the five subscales and a total score. Internal consistency reliability ranges from alpha = .90 for positive family affect to alpha = .74 for family conflicts (Tavitian et al., 1987).

Data Analysis

Descriptive analyses were conducted across the entire sample, followed by *t*-tests and chi square analyses to test for significant differences between the two shelter samples. Pearson correlations were conducted to identify PTSD scores associated with youth and family factors. Significant variables in these analyses were assessed using multiple regression to determine the predictors of adolescents' PTSD symptoms, while controlling for significant group differences.

RESULTS

Sample Demographics & Group Differences

The overall sample ($N = 350$) averaged about 15 years of age and were predominately female (see Table 1). The youth were primarily white (42.1%) or African American (37.7%) and nearly half (45.9%) had been living with

TABLE 1 Sample Characteristics

Demographics	Total sample $N = 350$	New York $n = 155$ (%)	Texas $n = 195$ (%)	χ^2
Gender				0.02
Male	154 (44.1)	69 (44.5)	85 (43.8)	
Female	195 (55.9)	86 (55.5)	109 (56.2)	
Ethnicity				28.39**
European American	147 (42.1)	61 (39.4)	86 (44.3)	
African American	132 (37.7)	76 (49.0)	56 (28.9)	
Hispanic	36 (10.3)	14 (9.0)	22 (11.3)	
American Indian	9 (2.6)	3 (1.9)	6 (3.1)	
Asian	3 (0.9)	1 (0.6)	2 (1.0)	
Mixed	22 (6.3)	0 (0.0)	22 (11.3)	
Living situation before admission				15.78**
parent's home	158 (45.9)	78 (50.3)	80 (42.3)	
adult relative/friend	130 (37.8)	56 (36.1)	74 (39.2)	
foster home	15 (4.4)	6 (3.9)	9 (4.8)	
institutional program	20 (5.8)	7 (4.5)	13 (6.9)	
street/temporary situation	21 (6.2)	6 (3.9)	13 (6.9)	
Expelled from school	153 (43.9)	88 (56.8)	65 (33.5)	32.9**
Youth reported neglect	77 (22.1)	47 (30.3)	74 (37.9)	12.3**
Youth reported being physically abused	79 (22.6)	24 (15.5)	55 (28.4)	−2.50*
Youth reported being sexually abused	31 (8.9)	4 (2.6)	27 (13.9)	−3.30**
	Mean (SD)	Mean (SD)	Mean (SD)	t-test
Age	15.3 (1.7)	16.0 (1.5)	14.8 (1.7)	7.07**
Number of times ran away	4.9 (11.8)	3.4 (3.5)	6.1 (15.6)	−1.97*
PTSD total score	68.4 (10.3)	69.8 (10.3)	67.3 (10.13)	2.31*

*$p \leqslant .05$, **$p \leqslant .01$.

parents at the time they ran away and were admitted to the youth emergency shelter. Youths' reported running away an average of 5 times ($SD \pm 11.8$) and had been away from home more than 5 days (mean = 5.52, SD 17.1). More than half of the respondents indicated they had ever smoked cigarettes (61.6%), drank alcohol (60.2%), or used marijuana (54.5%).

Chi-square and *t*-tests indicated some significant differences between runaway/homeless youths from Texas and New York. As shown in Table 1, the average age of New York youths was significantly greater than those in Texas, but the proportion of males and females was similar between the

TABLE 2 Single-Order Correlations of PTSD Symptoms with Youth and Family Factors

	Posttraumatic stress	
Independent variables	*r*	<*p*
Demographics		
Age	.03	.59
Gender	−.27	.001
Ethnicity	−.13	.01
Youth factors		
Substance use		
Ever use cigarettes	.04	.42
Ever use alcohol	.03	.64
Ever use marijuana	.04	.48
Ever use LSD	.12	.03
Ever use ecstasy	.08	.16
Ever use downers	.13	.02
Ever use uppers	.12	.04
Ever use inhalants	.17	.003
Health status	−.13	.02
Number of runaway episodes	−.01	.87
Poor academic performance	.15	.005
Depression	.73	.001
Anxiety	.72	.001
Dissociation	.69	.001
Anger	.54	.001
Sexual concerns	.23	.001
Family factors		
Father's substance use		
Marijuana use frequency	.12	.08
Ecstasy use frequency	.02	.96
LSD use frequency	.05	.45
Mother's substance use		
Marijuana use frequency	.14	.03
Ecstasy use frequency	.19	.004
LSD use frequency	.14	.03
Family member sexually abused youth	.14	.01
Family member physically abused youth	.16	.002
Family Functioning		
Worries	.25	.001
Communication	−.12	.03
Conflict	.24	.001

TABLE 3 Multiple Regression Model to Predict Posttraumatic Stress Scores

Variable	B	SE B	β	$<p$
Demographics				
Gender	−.81	1.39	−.04	.56
Ethnicity	.06	.30	.01	.84
Youth factors				
Substance use				
Ever use LSD	.99	1.80	.03	.58
Ever use downers	−2.40	1.99	−.06	.23
Ever use inhalants	−.83	1.82	−.02	.65
Health status	.90	.59	.07	.13
Poor academic performance	.84	1.11	.03	.45
Depression	.25	.07	.26	.001
Anxiety	.23	.07	.24	.002
Dissociation	.34	.08	.33	.000
Anger	.01	.07	.01	.88
Sexual concerns	.01	.02	.02	.68
Family factors				
Mother's ecstasy use	5.89	1.86	.21	.002
Mother's LSD use	−3.29	1.53	−.14	.03
Mother's marijuana use	.69	.63	.05	.27
Sexually abused youth	.14	1.56	.00	.93
Physically abused youth	.14	.42	.02	.74
Family Functioning				
Worries	.13	.05	.12	.016
Communication	−.14	.04	−.15	.001
Conflict	−.04	.05	−.04	.43

Note. Overall model $F(20, 201) = 20.10$, $p < .01$.
Adjusted $R^2 = .69$.

two groups. Ethnic differences were significant between the two groups; the greatest difference was in the proportion of African-American youths (49% in New York and 29% in Texas). A greater proportion of youths from New York reported living primarily with parents at the time of admission to the shelter, whereas a greater percentage of youths from Texas reported living on the streets or in a temporary situation before admission.

The runaway/homeless youth participants had an average score on the PTSD measure of 68.4 ($SD \pm 10.3$). Raw scores were transformed into standardized scores to indicate a mean of 50 and a standard deviation of 10. Scores above 65 are considered clinically significant as they equal or exceed 94% of the 'standardized sample' (Briere, 1996). Therefore, this score indicates elevated PTSD symptoms as compared to scale norms.

Factors Associated with PTSD Symptoms

Bivariate correlations were conducted to determine demographic, youth and family factors associated with PTSD. As shown in Table 2, PTSD was significantly associated with youth factors, including being male, European American, using LSD, 'downers', 'uppers', and inhalants, reporting poor health, and poor academic performance. Those with higher levels of depression, anxiety, dissociation, anger, and sexual concerns also had significantly higher rates of PTSD symptoms. Family factors associated with PTSD included mother's marijuana, LSD, and ecstasy use and the youth being physically or sexually abused in the home. Youth who reported feeling worried about family relationships, experienced less communication or more conflict in the family had higher PTSD scores.

Impact of Factors on PTSD Symptoms

Table 3 presents the results of the simultaneous multiple regression on PTSD symptom scores. Only scores on depression, anxiety, and dissociation, mother's ecstasy or LSD use, feeling worried about family relationships, and reporting poor family communication were significantly related to higher PTSD scores, $F(20, 201) = 20.10, p < .001$. This model accounted for 69% of the adjusted variance in the adolescent's PTSD scores.

DISCUSSION

The findings of this study of runaway/homeless youths in two areas of the country demonstrate the heightened rates of PTSD symptoms found among this highly vulnerable population. The average rates of PTSD symptoms in this group of adolescents were nearly twenty points higher than standardized averages developed for use with the TSCC scale (Briere, 1996); more than 98% had scores above 50, the standardized mean. Although these scores cannot be used to diagnose PTSD, the rates are substantially greater than epidemiological studies that indicate PTSD rates of 9.2% in young adults (Breslau, 2002) and 6.3% in older adolescents (Giaconia, Reinherz, Silverman, & Pakiz, 1995).

Depression, Anxiety, and Dissociation

PTSD symptom scores were significantly related to the psychological issues of depression, anxiety, and dissociation. These findings are similar to previous research of 18 year old adolescents who had experienced trauma, as these youth had behavioral and emotional problems, interpersonal problems, academic failure, depressive and suicidal behavior, and physical health problems (Giaconia et al., 1995). Other studies have shown strong associations between trauma and symptoms of depression and anxiety (Pine & Cohen, 2002; Stewart et al., 2004) and trauma experiences often predict increased risk for depression and anxiety (Breslau, 2002; Pynoos et al.,

1987; Steinberg & Avenevoli, 2000). As considerable research has linked measures of depressive symptoms to early family stresses (Conger et al., 1992,1993; Ge, Lorenz, Conger, Elder, & Simons, 1994), these findings suggest that traumatic or stressful life events are associated with a range of psychological symptoms. For youth who have experienced psychological distress related to traumatic experiences before they run away, the experience of running away likely exacerbates those symptoms. Thus, services to runaway/homeless youth need to more specifically assess and identify these symptoms. While youth shelters services are limited in dealing with these issues, offering appropriate referral sources is critical to the psychological health of these youth.

Substance Use

Substance use is also highly prevalent among this group of runaway/homeless youth; comparable to other studies of runaway/homeless youth (Kipke, Montgomery, Simon, & Iverson, 1997; Thompson, Maguin, & Pollio, 2003). The majority of youth reported using illicit substances; 60% drank alcohol, 55% smoked marijuana, and 11% used LSD. The higher rates of substance use among these youth is particularly problematic as drug use is often a significant pathway into adolescent homelessness and has been identified as a major obstacle for adolescents trying to get off the streets (MacLean, Paradise et al., 1999). Previous research has shown that injection drug using youth more frequently report traumatic psychosocial histories than non-injecting youth (Martinez et al., 1998). Thus, the extremely stressful and unstable living environments of runaway/homeless youths make PTSD symptoms much more likely. Although none of the substances remained significant predictors of PTSD symptom scores in this study, these findings suggest that runaway/homeless youth who use more hard-core substances, such as LSD, inhalants, amphetamines, and benzodiazepines report greater levels of PTSD symptoms. Interestingly, alcohol and marijuana use were not related to PTSD. It may be that these substances are so commonly used that they do not reflect a special circumstance in the manifestation of PTSD symptoms.

On the other hand, parental use (more specifically, the mother's use) of substances was significantly related to and predicted PTSD symptom scores. There is general agreement that parental alcoholism has disruptive and negative effects on family relationships and functioning (Sher, Gershuny, Peterson, & Raskin, 1997). Previous research reports that children of alcohol and drug users are at increased risk for abuse and neglect and that the reduced parental supervision that often accompanies drug use behaviors may leave the child vulnerable to other sources of victimization (Kilpatrick et al., 2000; Widom, 1993). Childhood stressors (e.g., disrupted family rituals, embarrassment, neglect, abuse) have been shown to be strongly related to a family history of substance use (Sher et al., 1997). In addition, studies have suggested that parental warmth and support (often lacking among parents of runaway/homeless youth) buffers the influence of negative life events on adolescents' mental-health trajectories (Ge et al., 1994). Thus, a mother's substance use may be an indicator of family dysfunction that has a profound negative influence on a youth's trauma symptomology.

The findings of this study suggest that runaway/homeless youth entering emergency shelters services must be evaluated concerning trauma and associated comorbid symptoms. Shelters currently evaluate youth through nonstandardized assessment measures and methods; standardized assessment techniques must be implemented if further understanding of the issues of this high-risk group of youth is to be developed. A variety of methods have been proposed to assess these issues, such as rigid, algorithm-structured approaches (Shaffer, Fisher, Lucas, Dulcan, & Schwab-Stone, 2000) or extensive training of workers in less structured approaches (Angold & Costello, 2000). Regardless of how these assessments are actually carried out, adolescent development and the context of their family environment must be recognized.

In addition, assessments much take into account the numerous barriers for youth to disclose their traumatic events to others. If a parent is the cause of the trauma, the youth may be reluctant to disclose the information to another adult (Cohen, 2003). Although some aspects of PTSD symptoms may be best reported by the youth themselves, other observers may provide additional objective descriptions of the youth's behavior (March, 2003). Those who work with adolescents should not underestimate the potential of a wide range of traumatic events that provoke PTSD symptoms, including those not involving direct violence or physical harm. Investigating the traumatic event(s) that lead to the development of PTSD symptoms, such as the youth's characteristics and family environments must be considered (Giaconia et al., 1995; MacLean, Embry, & Cauce, 1999).

LIMITATIONS

It is important to keep in mind the limitations of this study when reviewing the results. Although the two groups of youths were recruited to provide homogeneous and comparable samples, it should be noted that youth participants were from disparate regions of the country. Although both agencies were federally-funded shelters with comparable programs, some programmatic disparity is inevitable and cannot be accounted for in this study. The samples, however, appear to be unbiased as demographics of youths in this study are similar to statistics of youths using federally funded shelters nationwide (Thompson et al., 2003).

This study also relied on symptom inventories (e.g., Trauma Symptom Checklist for Children) rather than truly diagnostic assessments and the data were youth self-reports that cannot be independently verified. Thus, the information and the subject's reliability may be in question, which raises questions concerning these findings. Adolescent participants may have under-reported various characteristics they believe have a negative connotation (Safyer, Thompson, Maccio, Zittel-Palamra, & Forehand, in press), such as sexual or physical abuse, neglect, or substance use. Thus, these high-risk behaviors may be more extensive and problematic than reflected in the results. Finally, this study employed a cross-sectional design. While this approach is helpful in identifying possible variables for use in causal modeling, they cannot establish causal sequences. For example, it is impossible to discern if depression predates PTSD symptoms or visa versa.

Although generalization of the results of this study must be made with caution, the findings address a gap in the literature concerning runaway/homeless youths' trauma symptoms. Further studies with this population of adolescents are needed that incorporate longitudinal designs in order to capture trauma symptoms and the comorbid psychological consequences. There are few studies of the long-term outcomes of traumatic events among adults and even fewer of children and adolescents (Yule et al., 2000); thus future research is needed that focuses on the longitudinal issues associated with adolescent traumatic experiences. This information would be useful for devising sensitive assessment tools and subsequent interventions strategies for these high-risk adolescents.

ACKNOWLEDGEMENTS

The author gratefully acknowledges the youth shelter directors and staff who supported and assisted in this research and Kim Zittel-Palamara and Erin Snell who were instrumental in data collection.

REFERENCES

American Psychiatric Association. (1994). *Diagnostic and statistical manual of mental disorders* (4th ed.). Washington, DC: Author.

Angold, A. and Costello, E. J. (2000). The Child and Adolescent Psychiatric Assessment (CAPA). *Journal of American Academy of Child and Adolescent Psychiatry, 39*, 39–48.

Baer, J. S., Ginzler, J. A., and Peterson, P. L. (2003). DSM-IV alcohol and substance abuse and dependence in homeless youth. *Journal of Studies on Alcohol, 64*(1), 5–14.

Berkman, L. and Kawachi, I. (2000). *A historical framework for social epidemiology.* New York: Oxford University Press.

Breslau, N. (2002). Psychiatric morbidity in adult survivors of childhood trauma. *Seminar in Clinical Neuropsychiatry, 7*, 66–79.

Briere, J. (1996). *Trauma Symptoms Checklist for Children (TSCC): Professional manual*. Lutz, FL: Psychological Assessment Resources, Inc.

Cohen, D. A. (2003). Treating acute posttraumatic reactions in children and adolescents. *Society of Biological Psychiatry, 53*, 827–833.

Conger, R. D., Conger, K. J., Elder, G. H., Jr., Lorenz, F. O., Simmons, R. L., and Whitbeck, L. B. (1992). A family process model of economic hardship and adjustment of early adolescent boys. *Child Development, 63*(3), 526–541.

Conger, R. D., Conger, K. J., Elder, G. H., Lorenz, F. O., Simons, R. L., and Whitbeck, L. B. (1993). Family economic stress and adjustment of early adolescent girls. *Developmental Psychology, 29*(2), 206–219.

Crespi, T. D. and Sabatelli, R. M. (1993). Adolescent runaways and family strife: A conflict-induced differentiation framework. *Adolescence, 28*(112), 867–878.

Dadds, M. R., Braddock, D., Cuers, S., Elliott, A., and Kelly, A. (1993). Personal and family distress in homeless adolescents. *Community Mental Health Journal, 29*(5), 413–422.

Downey, G. and Walker, E. (1992). Distinguishing family-level and child-level influences on the development of depression and aggression in children at risk. *Development & Psychopathology, 4*(1), 81–95.

Farrow, J. A., Deisher, R. W., Brown, R., Kulig, J. W., and Kipke, M. D. (1992). Health and health needs of homeless and runaway youth. A position paper of the Society for Adolescent Medicine. *Journal of Adolescent Health, 13*(8), 717–726.

Forst, M. L. (1994). A substance use profile of delinquent and homeless youths. *Journal of Drug Education, 24*(3), 219–231.

Ge, X., Lorenz, F. O., Conger, R. D., Elder, G. H., and Simons, R. L. (1994). Trajectories of stressful life events and depressive symptoms during adolescence. *Developmental Psychology, 30*(4), 467–483.

Giaconia, R. M., Reinherz, H. Z., Silverman, A. B., and Pakiz, B. (1995). Traumas and posttraumatic stress disorder in a community population of older adolescents. *Journal of the American Academy of Child & Adolescent Psychiatry, 34*(10), 1369–1380.

Green, A. H. (1993). Child sexual abuse: Immediate and long term effects and intervention. *Journal of the American Academy of Child & Adolescent Psychiatry, 32*, 890–902.

Greene, J. M., Ennett, S. T., and Ringwalt, C. L. (1999). Prevalence and correlates of survival sex among runaway and homeless youth. *American Journal of Public Health, 89*(9), 1406–1409.

Greene, J. M. and Ringwalt, C. L. (1997). Substance use among runaway and homeless youth in three national samples. *American Journal of Public Health, 87*(2), 229–236.

Janus, M.-D., Archambault, F. X., Brown, S. W., and Welsh, L. A. (1995). Physical abuse in Canadian runaway adolescents. *Child Abuse & Neglect, 19*(4), 433–447.

Johnston, L. D., O'Malley, P. M., and Bachman, J. G. (2002). *Demographic subgroup trends for various licit and illicit drugs, 1975–2001*. Retrieved March 24th, 2004, from http://monitoringthefuture.org

Kilpatrick, D. G., Acierno, R., Saunders, B., Resnick, H. S., Best, C. L., and Schnurr, P. P. (2000). Risk factors for adolescent substance abuse and dependence: Data from a national sample. *Journal of Consulting and Clinical Psychology, 68*(1), 19–30.

Kipke, M. D., Montgomery, S. B., Simon, T. R., and Iverson, E. F. (1997). "Substance abuse" disorders among runaway and homeless youth. *Substance Use & Misuse, 32*(7–8), 969–986.

Lifson, A. R. and Halcón, L. L. (2001). Substance abuse and high-risk needle related behaviors among homeless youth in Minneapolis: Implications for prevention. *Journal of Urban Health, 78*(4), 690–698.

MacLean, M. G., Embry, L. E., and Cauce, A. M. (1999). Homeless adolescents' paths to separation from family: Comparison of family characteristics, psychological adjustment, and victimization. *Journal of Community Psychology, 27*(2), 179–187.

MacLean, M. G., Paradise, M. J., and Cauce, A. M. (1999). Substance use and psychological adjustment in homeless adolescents: A test of three models. *American Journal of Community Psychology, 27*(3), 405–427.

March, J. S. (2003). Acute stress disorder in youth: A multivariate prediction model. *Society of Biological Psychiatry, 53*, 809–816.

Martinez, T. E., Gleghorn, A., Marx, R., Clements, K., Boman, M., and Katz, M. H. (1998). Psychosocial histories, social environment, and HIV risk behaviors of injection and noninjection drug using homeless youths. *Journal of Psychoactive Drugs, 30*(1), 1–10.

Mundy, P., Robertson, M., Robertson, J., and Greenblatt, M. (1990). The prevalence of psychotic symptoms in homeless adolescents. *Journal of the American Academy of Child and Adolescent Psychiatry, 29*(5), 724–731.

Pynoos, R. S., Frederick, C., Nader, K., Arroyo, W., Steinberg, A., and Eth, S. et al. (1987). Life threat and posttraumatic stress in school-age children. *Archives of General Psychiatry, 44*(12), 1057–1063.

Richters, J. E. (1993). Community violence and children's development: Toward a research agenda for the 1990s. *Psychiatry, 56*(1), 3–6.

Ringwalt, C. L., Greene, J. M., and Robertson, M. J. (1998). Familial backgrounds and risk behaviors of youth with thrownaway experiences. *Journal of Adolescence, 21*(3), 241–252.

Ringwalt, C. L., Greene, J. M., Robertson, M., and McPheeters, M. (1998). The prevalence of homelessness among adolescents in the United States. *American Journal of Public Health, 88*(9), 1325–1329.

Rotheram-Borus, M. J. (1993). Suicidal behavior and risk factors among runaway youths. *American Journal of Psychiatry, 150*(1), 103–107.

Safyer, A. E., Thompson, S., Maccio, E., Zittel-Palamra, K., and Forehand, G. (in press). Adolescent and parent perceptions of runaway behavior: Problems and solutions. *Child and Adolescent Social Work Journal.*

Shaffer, D., Fisher, P., Lucas, C. P., Dulcan, M. K., and Schwab-Stone, M. E. (2000). NIMH Diagnostic Interview Schedule for Children Version IV (NIMH DISC-IV): Description, differences from previous versions, and reliability of some common diagnoses. *Journal of American Academy of Child and Adolescent Psychiatry, 93*, 28–38.

Sher, K. J., Gershuny, B. S., Peterson, L., and Raskin, G. (1997). The role of childhood stressors in the intergenerational transmission of alcohol use disorders. *Journal of Studies on Alcohol, 58*(4), 414–427.

Steinberg, L. and Avenevoli, S. (2000). The role of context in the development of psychopathology: A conceptual framework and some speculative propositions. *Child Development, 71*(1), 66–74.

Stewart, A. J., Steiman, M., Cauce, A. M., Cochran, B. N., Whitbeck, L. B., and Hoyt, D. R. (2004). Victimization and posttraumatic stress disorder among homeless adolescents. *Child & Adolescent Social Work Journal, 21*(1), 325–331.

Tavitian, M., Lubiner, J. L., Green, L., Grebstein, L. C., and Velicer, W. F. (1987). Dimensions of family functioning. *Journal of Social Behavior and Personality, 2*, 191–204.

Thompson, S. J., Maguin, E., and Pollio, D. E. (2003). National and regional differences among runaway youth using federaly funded crisis shelters. *Journal of Social Service Research, 30*(1), 1–17.

Whitbeck, L. B. and Hoyt, D. R. (1999). *Nowhere to go: Homeless and runaway adolescents and their families.* New York: Aldine De Gruyter.

Whitbeck, L. B. and Hoyt, D. R. (2000). Depressive symptoms and co-occurring depressive symptoms, substance abuse, and conduct problems among runaway and homeless adolescents. *Child Development, 71*(3), 721–732.

Whitbeck, L. B., Hoyt, D. R., and Ackley, K. A. (1997). Abusive family backgrounds and later victimization among runaway and homeless adolescents. *Journal of Research on Adolescence, 7*(4), 375–392.

Whitbeck, L. B. and Simons, R. L. (1990). Life on the streets. The victimization of runaway and homeless adolescents. *Youth & Society, 22*(1), 108–125.

Widom, C. S. (1993). *Child abuse and alcohol use and abuse* (No. NIAAA Research Monograph No. 24, NIH Publication No 93-3496). Rockville, MD: Department of Health and Human Services.

Williams, N. R., Lindsey, E. W., Kurtz, P., and Jarvis, S. (2001). From trauma to resiliency: Lessons from former runaway and homeless youth. *Journal of Youth Studies, 4*(2), 233–253.

Yule, W., Bolton, D., Udwin, O., Boyle, S., O'Ryan, D., and Nurrish, J. (2000). The long-term psychological effects of a disaster experienced in adolescence: I: The incidence and course of PTSD. *Journal of Child Psychology & Psychiatry & Allied Disciplines, 41*(4), 503–511.

6

"I Came to Prison to Do My Time — Not to Get Raped": Coping Within the Institutional Setting

SHERYL PIMLOTT KUBIAK, JULIE HANNA, and
MARIANNE BALTON

Wayne State University, Detroit, MI, USA

Rarely is trauma discussed in relation to incarceration — either prison as a site of new trauma, the effect of incarceration on those with trauma histories, or the effect of trauma-related disorders on recidivism. This is particularly troublesome given the relationship between posttraumatic stress disorder

(PTSD) and substance use disorders (SUD; see Stewart, Ouimette, & Brown, 2003), and the high prevalence of SUD among women involved in the criminal justice system. Furthermore, substance use and abuse have clearly been key contributing factors to the significant increase in incarceration, particularly among women.

Women's trauma exposure prior to prison is likely to entail physical and/or sexual assault. Similar exposure may also occur during incarceration. International human rights groups have illuminated the incidence of abuses such as rape, molestation, sexual harassment, improper search and surveillance procedures and retaliation for reporting, most often implicating male staff (Amnesty International, 1999; Human Rights Watch, 1996). This abuse has been substantiated through congressional inquiry (U.S. General Accounting Office, 1999) and litigation in several states, with courts awarding monetary damages and mandating reform (LaBelle, 2002). Unfortunately, there has been a lack of attention to the effects of such abuse on the mental health and substance-use behaviors of women (both during and after incarceration) or to the coping methods women employ within the confines of the institution.

Accordingly, our descriptive analysis used case studies to examine women's experiences of prison-based victimization and the ways in which they cope within the institutional setting. Because a systematic assessment of the abuse in women's prisons was unlikely for several reasons,[1] we relied on secondary data collected as part of an investigation and later used in a class action lawsuit on behalf of the affected women. The evidence introduced for the litigation is public record and as such, we were able to conduct a review of histories, incident reports, personal reactions and psychological assessments. The goal of the paper was twofold: 1) to provide a descriptive assessment of the women's experiences through the use of case narrative and 2) to examine how context (e.g. prison) may affect coping strategies.

BACKGROUND

The United States has the highest rate of incarceration in the world, both in general and specifically that of females. Between 1980 and 1994, the number of women entering State and Federal prisons increased by 386%, as compared to 214% for men (Bureau of Justice Statistics, 1994). This growth has been precipitated by the "War on Drugs," which accounted for an 888% increase in the number of women incarcerated for drug offenses between 1985 and 1996 (Mauer, Potler, & Wolf, 1999). Nationally, 63% of women test positive for an illegal drug at the time of arrest, while 42% meet criteria for a diagnosis of drug dependence (National Institute of Justice, 2003). Rates of current SUD among incarcerated women range from 30–52% for drugs and 17–25% for alcohol disorders (Jordan, Schlenger, Fairbank, & Caddell, 1996; Teplin, Abram, & McClelland, 1996).

A disproportionate number of incarcerated women are young, poor, and of minority status; often they have limited education and have been responsible for the care of minor children prior to their confinement (Pimlott & Sarri, 2002). Approximately 40% of women worked full-time prior to arrest and over half (56%) have completed high school or obtained a general equivalency diploma. Minority women are more likely to serve time in jail or prison, in contrast to White women, who have a greater likelihood of being put on probation (Greenfeld & Snell, 1999).

Perhaps more significant to this study are the histories of sexual/physical abuse, the high prevalence of mental health issues (including trauma-related disorders) and SUD. Incarcerated women are almost four times as likely to be physically or sexually abused before prison as compared to their male counterparts (Morash, Bynum, & Koons, 1998). Women involved in the criminal justice system have higher rates of psychiatric disorders than women in the surrounding geographic areas (Jordan et al., 1996; Teplin et al., 1996) and similarly higher rates of SUD and other psychosocial stressors than other groups of impoverished women (Kubiak, Siefert, & Boyd, 2004). A recent assessment of all women incarcerated within this particular state system found that 70% were drug dependent. Furthermore, among females in State prisons, almost half were under the influence of drugs or alcohol at the time of arrest; 60% reported using drugs in the month prior to arrest; and nearly a third said they committed the offense in order to obtain money to support their need for drugs (Greenfeld & Snell, 1999).

A history of trauma not only has implications for consequent substance use, but conversely, substance use disorders place individuals at higher risk for victimization and abuse. Trauma, mental health, and substance use are all part of an interconnected cycle, in which each is potentially influenced by the other two. Individuals with co-occurring trauma-related disorders and substance abuse tend to use cocaine and opiates, the most severe substances; this is likely due to the use of substances as a form of self-medication to cope with the pain of previous trauma (Breslau, Davis, Peterson, & Schultz, 1997; Cottler, Compton, Mager, Spitznagel, & Janca, 1992). Furthermore, these individuals are more vulnerable to repeated trauma and victimization than individuals with substance abuse alone (Dansky, Brady, & Saladin, 1998).

Prison Environment

Since the colonial era, women have been incarcerated with or supervised by men, and subjected to sexual coercion and abuse by male custodians (Belknap, 2001; Morash & Schram, 2002). To address the exploitation and sexual abuse of incarcerated females, nineteenth century social reformers called for separate institutions, and in 1873 the first institution with an all female staff was founded (Morash & Schram, 2002). Female-staffed facilities remained the norm until the latter part of the 20th century when various legal challenges were supported by equal employment opportunity rights under Title VII. In the 1990s, reports of sexually degrading treatment of female prisoners began to surface as women complained of sexualized comments about their bodies, molestation that was officially referred to as a security 'pat down,' and forced sex (Kubiak, Boyd, Slayden & Young, in press).

This environment of 'total control' is characteristic of most closed institutional settings and may compound the psychological consequences of abuse (See Kubiak, in press). Closed organizations, such as residential care facilities, children's homes and prisons, are relatively isolated from the outside world, and as such, violations and violence are often contained and intensified (Hearn & Parkin, 2001). "Closed organizations or total institutions involve the total or attempted control of bodies of residents, including their sexuality, as people eat, sleep, work, and play under a unified organizational structure" (Hearn & Parkin, p. 105). Those living within these total institutions are often stigmatized and have no voice. In fact, in these settings, "Residents can adapt or resist but have little chance of being believed" (p. 117). Prisoners often adapt or cope, with a de facto code of silence regarding abuse during incarceration in order to protect themselves from further stigmatization (Heney & Kristiansen, 1997).

Coping

Coping strategies are conscious and purposeful efforts to reduce stress and reality are frequently clustered as either adaptive or maladaptive. Adaptive coping, usually operationalized as action-oriented, problem/solution-focused behavior, involves engaged responses that resolve or remove the source of stress, unlike maladaptive or emotion-focused coping, which provides temporary escape or avoidance through disengagement (see Compas, Connor-Smith, Saltzman, Thomsen, & Wadsworth, 2001, for review). Adaptive problem-focused coping has been linked to more favorable outcomes (Folkman & Lazarus, 1980, 1985; Pearlin, Menaghan, & Lieberman, 1981) compared with emotion-focused coping (i.e., praying, avoidance, use of drugs or alcohol), which is considered passive and usually ineffective (Compas et al., 2000; Banyard & Graham-Bermann, 1993).

Women in disempowered positions experience a compromised range of options for coping (Landrine & Klonoff, 1996). For example, Fine (1984) assessed the options available to a rape survivor, who was also an impoverished woman of color, illuminating how appraisal and coping strategies are evaluated within context. The woman believed that reporting the assault to authorities (active coping) would result in retaliation and subsequent harm to her family, and therefore enlisted various emotion-focused strategies, such as avoidance, to cope with the situation. The coping repertoire was dependent upon the available options and represented a variation of instrumentality. Lykes' (1983) study of African-American women coping with discrimination demonstrated that choice of coping strategies was dependent upon the environmental context of the discrimination. Those in predominantly Black organizations tended to use active coping compared with those in White organizations who used passive techniques. Similarly, Kaiser, and Miller (2004) found that women were much less likely to confront sexist behavior if there were high personal costs.

Thus, emotion-focused coping may be utilized to solve problems under conditions in which problem-focused coping will be ineffectual, or more pointedly, as a survival strategy (Banyard & Graham-Bermann, 1993; Freyd, 1996; Morrow & Smith, 1995). Thus environmental context, in this case the prison, must be considered in any examination of coping.

Reactions to encounters or stressors are dependent upon an individual's appraisal of what that encounter implies for his/her personal well-being (Smith & Lazarus, 1989). That is, events hold meaning based on prior knowledge, beliefs, and experiences that are unique to the individual. Therefore, an individual's appraisal of an event is a product of both the environmental context and individual history. While appraisal is the cognitive process of evaluating a situation, coping is defined as the cognitive and behavioral efforts to master, tolerate, or reduce external and internal demands and conflicts. Appraisal of the stressor is linked to the choice of coping response in any specific situation.

Current Study

The current study focused on three women's experiences of harassment and/or assault during incarceration, illuminating their experiences of the institutional environment and the coping strategies enlisted by each woman—and more importantly the choices of coping strategies available to them. The study described each woman's history prior to incarceration, her perception of the event and her appraisal of the situation. The use of case narratives allowed each woman to explain her story and her reasons for selecting specific coping strategies. These case narratives were framed within a very specific situation to address the following question: How do women cope with sexual harassment and abuse in a closed institutional setting?

METHOD

Case studies have often been used to provide in-depth analyses of persons within specified contexts, and to understand the extent to which context shapes the lives of individuals (Gilgun, 2001). In contrast to quantitative methods, the case study highlights how a context impacts individual units of study.

Narrative case studies are often used to highlight the therapeutic relationship between client and therapist, integrating the "historically important dynamic issues that might have relevance to the clients presenting symptomology" (Brandell & Vargas, 2001). A narrative analysis is a means by which the individual conveys meaning through use of his/her personal story and experience allowing for shifting connections between past, present and future (Riessman, 2001).

This narrative case study is unique because rather than describing a clinical relationship with one client, it focuses on the stories of three women using two sources of secondary data: case records and video depositions. We chose secondary data because of its unobtrusive nature, while retaining the individual's 'voice.' Because the women had been subject to multiple lines of inquiry related to the abuse, the secondary data allowed us to reinterpret existing data for alternative purposes (Krysik, 2001). In addition, using secondary analysis allowed us to include more than one type of data (i.e., micro-level, aggregate-level, or qualitative-level) in order to facilitate a more thorough understanding of these particular cases (Gilgun, 2001). Although access to the secondary data through court records did not require participant consent, per the institutional review board, we did request permission from the involved women.

The analysis began with a review of general case materials, such as plaintiff and defense positions, expert testimony, and case descriptors on all of the 32 women involved in the class action. Based on this overview, we purposefully selected three cases that were representative of the types of offenses litigated in the case and demographics of the women involved in the criminal justice system. After selecting the cases, we chose to focus on coping because of the unique environmental context and concerns as to the length of the paper.

In an effort to increase reliability of the group in defining coping strategies, we used categories and items from Folkman and Lazurus' (1980) Ways of Coping Scale. The eight subscales (i.e., confrontive, distancing, self-controlling, seeking social support, accepting responsibility, escape/avoidance, planful problem solving and positive reappraisal) reflect three larger domains: 1) problem-focused coping, 2) emotion-focused coping, and 3) seeking social support—conceptualized as problem-focused. Some of the coping strategies defined within the scale may be incongruent with the prison environment, hence we used the individual subscale definitions, as well as individual items, to define the larger categories of problem-focused (i.e., active) and emotion-focused (i.e., passive) coping.

Using this approach, we again examined the case files for evidence of coping strategies the women utilized while in prison. Team members discussed specific behaviors and defined them as either problem or emotion-focused coping. While there was some disagreement over the subscale categories subsumed by the broader categories, there was unanimous agreement on the broader categories, thus creating inter-rater reliability. We subsequently reviewed the video depositions to hear the women's explanations and understanding of specific behaviors.

RESULTS

Case 1: Monica—"I came to Prison to do my time, not to get raped"

According to a Department of Corrections (DOC) evaluation, Monica's[2] childhood was "chaotic" and "indisputabl(y)... less than idyllic." In fact, a 1990 court report stated, "Monica's whole life has been a series of sexual and physical abuse." Monica's mother was addicted to drugs and sometimes engaged in prostitution. Records in the juvenile court documented neglect by her mother, who was also physically and verbally abusive. Her mother had a series of boyfriends, and Monica was uncertain about which one was her biological father. One of these men, whom she believed to be her father, sexually abused her between the ages of 2 and 10, which resulted in his conviction of criminal sexual conduct (CSC). Two years later, Monica was sexually abused by her mother's new boyfriend, although her mother remained in a relationship with him.

In order to escape the abuse, Monica began running away from home when she was nine years old. Between the ages of 12 and 16, she was in and out of foster homes, often truanting, which led to a record of "repeated home desertion" with the juvenile court. By this time, she had already experimented with marijuana and was drinking heavily. She had also attempted suicide three times, the first attempt being at the age of five. In the ninth grade, Monica became pregnant, dropped out of school, and moved into her own apartment.

At the age of 16, Monica became the mother of a newborn son and still had no criminal record. However, within one month, she was arrested four times. While the first three charges of retail fraud and aggravated assault were pending against her, Monica was arrested with three males and one other female for being involved in a rape. Monica was drinking excessively on the night of the incident, reporting to police, "...I don't remember most of that night...I can't believe I did something like this all because of peer pressure and alcohol." Monica was convicted of first-degree CSC and sentenced to 20 to 30 years in prison.

While incarcerated, Monica was sexually assaulted by male guards on two separate occasions. The first incident occurred two years into her prison sentence, when an officer told Monica that she had not been with a man in a long time, and that she should be ready for him when he came back to her cell. Monica stated that he did not use physical force, nor did she fight or struggle as he raped her three times that night. She took her underwear off because "he told me to...If I don't follow a direct order, I can get a write-up for major misconduct." She did not want to report the assault for fear of retaliation; however, she talked about the incident to her therapist, who then reported it to authorities against Monica's will. Monica felt that the therapist betrayed her confidence by reporting the incident, after which time Monica was referred for psychiatric assessment. She presented with depression, anxiety, intrusive thoughts of the incident, and fear of loud noises, as well as feelings of helplessness and chronic pessimism. She described recurrent nightmares in which she was being raped by the perpetrator and was unable to move or defend herself. Monica felt that she was "cursed because others always seem to hurt me. Sometimes I just wish I were dead." However, she later minimized her symptoms by saying, "Oh really, it's OK now. I want to go back to [prison]." Furthermore, she claimed responsibility for the incident, stating, "I didn't say yes and I didn't say no. When he was comin' on to me before, I just laughed it off."

The following year, Monica was referred for a mental health evaluation again because of an increase in existing symptoms and negative feelings about herself, as well as loss of appetite and difficulty concentrating. She stated that could not sleep or eat, and wanted to get help before she "got sick again." In addition, she reported feeling socially withdrawn and irritable, and a fear that she would lose control and start a fight. The psychologist assessed that Monica perceived others as threatening to her, especially the guards. In fact, the perpetrator continued to send harassing messages to her even though he was off the housing unit. In addition, other officers threatened to send her to another part of the facility and taunted her by saying, "It's not a crime to rape a rapist. You deserved it."

Within a few months, another officer began harassing her with sexually-explicit language, and fondled her on one occasion. Shortly thereafter, he gave her condoms and told her that he wanted to have sex with her, which Monica "felt was real threatening." She stated that it was not a verbal or physical threat, but rather his demeanor. She did not resist taking the condoms because she was scared, and wanted to have protection in case he came back. She responded to this gesture as she did to previous sexual advances by thinking to herself or stating aloud, "Yeah, right. Whatever." She explained that this meant, "Whatever you say. It don't matter. Like I wasn't taking him serious. ... Deep in my heart, I was ... but I didn't want him to know he was intimidating me." Based on her experience related to the previous rape, she felt that, "Nobody is going to protect me. ... They didn't do nothing the first time." She did not report the officer for giving her condoms because she believed that she would get written up for "interfering with administrative rules." Instead, she kept the condoms on top of her desk, hoping that they would be discovered in a shakedown (search of her cell).

Later that night, Monica stated, "The officer came in, pulled me to the floor, and had sex with me." Again, she did not resist because she assumed that she would be accused of fighting, which would result in "catching a new case" and spending time in segregation. When asked to recount what the officer said when he was in her room, she stated, "I don't remember. I really wasn't paying no attention. It was kinda like I was really not there anymore ... I wasn't there." The officer left the condom on the floor, and Monica flushed it down the toilet. When asked why, she responded, "What else could I do with it? ... Other things ... wouldn't have worked....I was just gonna kill myself and get it over with." This time she did not tell anyone about the rape, but responded instead by overdosing on Haldol.

Monica was sent to an external mental-health facility for evaluation and treatment. By this time, Monica had become increasingly preoccupied with thoughts of death, and began to experience flashbacks of being raped as a child. She was consumed with fear that an officer would "come and get" her again. She reported a lack of control over her own body, stating, "I'm tired of people taking my body. ... If I don't give my body to people, they'll take it." However, she indicated feeling safer at the outside facility, resulting in improved sleep and appetite. In fact, she admitted that she was "doing those things [suicide attempts] to get away from there."

After her release from the mental-health facility, Monica was moved to another correctional site, where she continued to feel unsafe. In fact, she felt antagonized by the entire system: "I'm in a no-win situation. ... We're convicts and criminals, and no one cares. ... These men abuse women, but the system acts like it's nothing... When other women are raped, the men go to prison for life." She not only felt helpless to defend herself from being raped, she felt that she was at the mercy of the guards overall, explaining, "They always have the upper hand on you. You never know what they'll say or do." She even feared that after release she would have to "watch her back" and move from the state.

Monica avoided talking about the incidents because it increased the frequency of her nightmares. She did, however, keep a journal in which she wrote about the sexual assaults. She was careful not to mention the names of the offending officers for fear of "getting in trouble" if anyone ever read the journal. Because the journal included her "deepest thoughts," she felt violated when it was taken as evidence for court proceedings.

When describing how she currently felt, she stated, "I've been cheated. ...I feel real worthless. ...They use(d) their authority to get what they wanted." However, she began to display a desire to regain control after retaining legal counsel, as she stated, "It's time for me to stand up for myself. I'm not going to allow them to do just anything to me anymore...I do have say-so over my body." She also revealed that she was surprised to be holding up, stating, "I didn't think I'd be as strong as I am now."

Case 2: Rhonda—"Nobody's going to believe you—you're a convict"

As an infant, Rhonda was abandoned by her biological mother; when she was three years old, her father married the woman whom Rhonda came to regard as her mother. Rhonda described her as a 'mean drunk' who inflicted severe physical abuse. She described her father as loving, but absent, and was sexually abused by her half brother between the ages of 6 and 13. She completed high school and left home shortly thereafter to enter a vocational training program out of state. Although she completed training in computer processing, she returned to her home community and worked as a cocktail waitress, topless dancer, and in a massage parlor. She argued that she never sold herself for sex, but she posed as a prostitute in a scheme to rob would-be customers. She began drug use (cocaine) at the age of 24 and heavy use of crack cocaine ("a few hundred dollars per day") the following year. While she indicated multiple arrests (e.g., disorderly conduct, flagging, and accosting and soliciting), most did not result in formal charges. Her first felony conviction brought about a probation sentence, but a probation violation resulted in incarceration in the state prison. Since that time, she was in and out of prison, due to drugs and the inability to successfully complete probation or parole sentences.

Rhonda joined the lawsuit as a result of being sexually molested by an officer during the intake process in the quarantine unit. As prisoners entered the institution they were restricted to their cells 22 hours/day for approximately 30 days while various assessments were administered and processed by corrections staff. Rhonda stated that many of the officers were sexually gratified by the female inmates. One particular officer used to unlock her cell door, enter the room and say, "Assume the position." The 'position' is one that is used for a pat down, an over-the-clothes search of the body that requires an individual to stand with legs apart and arms fully extended to the sides. When the officer began fondling her and rubbing his genitals on her body, she asked him to stop. He laughed and said, "It's going to be your word against mine and nobody's going to believe you, you're a convict—look at your record." This particular officer came into her room "whenever he felt like it." Rhonda said that she kept the allegations to herself because she could not trust the system: "If the officer says it happened, then it happened. ... The police are not our friends. The ones I've encountered have made me leery of the rest."

Although she was fully aware of the grievance procedure, Rhonda decided not to tell anyone because "you don't file complaints if you want to go home." When asked if she told other inmates about her abuse she said, "I kept it to myself, close to my chest" as a way to circumvent harassment from other guards. Rhonda described a retaliatory system in which the perpetrating officer's colleagues would write "bogus" tickets to remind the women that the men were watching out for each other.

Rhonda relayed the events of an earlier confinement in which an officer who transported female prisoners to the work camp accosted her for oral sex, telling her that she would not go home if she did not perform. The officer threatened her by implying that he would write her a ticket for trying to run away from the work crew, saying, "Don't you have a center [parole] date?

They do prosecute escapees here." Rhonda complied on numerous occasions in order to avoid escape tickets, especially considering that her release was pending. She attempted to quit the work crew but was prohibited by the unit officer. When asked in the deposition if she reported it, she replied, "What do you say? It's my word against his."

This threat was especially poignant to Rhonda, as her current sentence was related to an escape ticket that she had received while at a community corrections center. During her stay at the center, which was a co-ed substance-abuse treatment program, she was involved in a sexual relationship with another resident. Because such relationships were strictly forbidden under the program's rules, she was told that she would be discharged from the program and returned to prison. Her fear of reincarceration prompted her to run away but she turned herself in 33 days later. She then learned that she would not have been returned to prison because of the program discharge, but would be returned on an 'escape' charge due to the 33-day absence.

Rhonda said that the assault experiences during her confinement left her feeling embarrassed, degraded, and humiliated. She had flashbacks of the incidents, and on one occasion reported a flashback as a result of watching a movie in which someone was sexually assaulted. Rhonda claimed that she had nightmares about the incidents, and in fact woke up screaming in anticipation of the deposition. She lost weight, often slept 18 hours a day and sobbed hysterically for no apparent reason. She saw the prison physician for severe headaches, which were diagnosed as stress-related. When asked why she did not report these symptoms to the prison psychologist, she said that she did not want to be put on medication: "If you're on medication, it holds up your parole. ... It doesn't look good to the parole board. ... You can't go to the center until you're off meds for over a year."

Case 3: June—"It's like he was in control of me"

June's history of mental-health treatment dates back to age four when she received counseling after her parents divorced. She resided with her father, a high-school teacher, who provided a more secure environment than her mother, a bar manager. June and her brother were raised in a strict but loving manner. Eventually, her father married a colleague who was ten years older than June. She claimed, "I was mouthy, stubborn, and strong willed, but not disrespectful," although she often rebelled against her stepmother's authority. June began to drink and smoke marijuana in order to fit in with her peers, as well as mitigate the negative feelings that she held toward her stepmother. As tensions increased, she decided to live with her mother. Despite her acting out, June considered her family a strong support system.

As a high-school student, June's drug and alcohol use escalated from marijuana and alcohol to the use of cocaine 3–4 times per week. An auto accident while she was under the influence of alcohol and marijuana resulted in several broken bones, internal bleeding, and a closed head injury. As a first offense, June received 90 days probation. She also received treatment for posttraumatic stress disorder, closed head injury, alcohol and drug abuse, and impulsive behavior. A short time afterward, June was raped by her boyfriend's best friend. Although she wanted to press charges, the prosecutor's office refused because she was drunk at the time.

Throughout these years, June was continually involved with treatment providers as well as the criminal justice system. She sought, or was mandated to, various mental-health and substance-abuse treatment programs, none of which she successfully completed. She had three suicide attempts, at ages 20, 21, and 23. June's legal record includes several arrests and convictions: vicious destruction of property, drunk and disorderly conduct, false statements to police, being a minor in possession of alcohol and drugs, forgery, retail fraud, shoplifting, possession of financial transaction devices, and for multiple tether and probation violations. One such probation violation resulted in a 6-month incarceration at the age 21, followed by a conviction for retail fraud. On the basis of repeated violations, her probation was finally revoked, and June was sentenced to 4 to 14 years in prison.

During her incarceration she felt betrayed and punished by the people whom she believed would protect her, including the staff, psychiatrist, and officers. Prison mental-health workers claimed that June was being manipulative by clinging to her illnesses and resisting all attempts at rehabilitation. The prison psychiatrist diagnosed June with possible epilepsy or dissociative disorder with borderline features.

June actively used the grievance procedure to report being illegally searched, harassed, and propositioned by officers. One officer gave her the choice to blow kisses to the other officers or scrub toilets; similarly, he harassed her while she made telephone calls. The majority of the harassment she endured came from the shift commander, whom she said, "made my life hell" because he used his authority to "scare the shit out of me." This shift commander frequently stood outside her cell door, glaring at her until she felt that he was "in control" of her and that "he was going to get me." He kept track of her activities by engaging officers to report "June citings" using their walkie-talkies, and speaking about her activities within earshot. He frequently questioned other inmates regarding her behavior, "making it sound like I was a paranoid, crazy person."

Early in her confinement, June informed two female officers about the commander's activities, hoping to document his misconduct. June realized that her complaints would be in vain as they explained to her that all complaints of harassment went to the shift commander. June reported that the shift commander retaliated by engaging his colleagues to "cover his ass" by issuing her tickets for slander and for interfering with administrative rules. Officers refused to accept subsequent complaints against the shift commander, asserting that she was a liar.

The first time the shift commander singled her out for extra duty June complied. Afterward, she inquired about any further instructions, to which he replied by staring at her genital area and asking what she thought. She reported, "The way he looked at me was degrading. He had a smirk on his face." This incident, June claims, marked the beginning of a relationship of constant harassment. She said, "He began with verbal bullshit," making comments "to break down my self-respect."

On another occasion, the shift commander requested that she clean his office, whereupon leaving, June asked if there was anything more she was required to do. The commander replied by looking at his groin, and suggested that the two of them could think of something. June again left the room without discussion. During a subsequent extra duty assignment the shift commander requested that June buff the floors of his office, which were carpeted. As she pointed out the impossibility of the task, the shift commander ordered her to jump on the desk and show him what she could do. June again responded by leaving the room without comment.

As a consequence, June received numerous citations for what she believes were fictitious infractions, which delayed her release for an additional nine months. June felt that this extended confinement was likewise the result of retaliation. At one point, she attempted to grieve the tickets, assisted by a family member who served as a judge in a neighboring county. Upon investigation, it was determined that her complaints were justified.

June's mother also made contact with the warden of the facility, who promised to investigate June's complaints but failed to follow through. Eventually, her mother contacted Internal Affairs who then informed June that because of her history of fraud, she was most likely being dishonest about the harassment.

Subsequent to this decision, and after receiving misconduct tickets in the two weeks prior to her parole hearing, June became fearful and followed her mother's advice to be compliant. The misconduct tickets yielded her four to five days of confinement to her room with no outside contact. She reported that this experience exacerbated her sense of anger, depression, frustration, and shame.

After release, June was fearful of returning to prison where she was demeaned, told that she was a liar, and felt the environment brought out her "hostile emotions." She felt that she "entered prison with low self-esteem" and was released "with worse self-esteem." June perceived the experience of incarceration as a time during which she was humiliated by teams of individuals—including mental health staff—who turned against her. June also currently complained of eating problems, and of having gained seventy-five pounds during the first year after release. She was angry with the shift commander and with the DOC for failing to protect her. She continued to experience insomnia, nightmares, cold sweats, flashbacks of harassment, anxiety, extreme stress when recalling events, and difficulties concentrating.

DISCUSSION

This paper explores the institutional environment that drug-involved women may encounter during incarceration; specifically, the paper uses a narrative case study approach to describe the stories of three women who experienced sexual assault and/or harassment during their incarcerations. Each of the women has a history of substance use and sexual/physical assault prior to incarceration. Likewise substance use contributed to the behaviors that pro-pelled each woman into the criminal justice system. While such histories have implications for post-release behavior, our focus is on the ways in which the women coped with abuse within the prison setting. Using second-ary data, we reconstructed their histories and events during incarceration without re-interviewing (or re-traumatizing) the women. Our goals are to illuminate the women's experiences; explore coping strategies as a mech-anism for achieving individual mental health, safety, and stability for those who remain confined in the institution post-abuse; and to suggest strategies for intervention during and after incarceration.

The case scenarios encapsulate a continuum of the types of abuse experienced during incarceration, the histories of abuse prior to incarcer-ation, the individual perceptions of available coping strategies, and the 'choices' of strategies utilized. Because the first three factors (i e., abuse type, prior history, and perceptions of options) are salient to the choice of coping strategies utilized, care should be taken not to generalize across cases or compare each woman's coping strategies. Overall, however, the prison environment does restrict opportunities for efficacious behaviors that might protect the women from abuse. Certainly, a woman cannot leave of her own volition, nor can she move freely about, choosing to live in one unit ver-sus another. In addition, the women depicted in these vignettes clearly describe how their attempts at self-protection were, or could be, interpreted by corrections staff as insolence or as threatening.

As we expected with the continuum of cases selected, there is variation among the women in the coping strategies enlisted. For example, only one woman made attempts to vocally confront and participate in the grievance process as a result of the harassment (June). Interestingly, this woman had a powerful outside network (e.g., her uncle was a judge), and may also have endured some cognitive deficits as a result of an earlier incident. After all of her own and her family's efforts at advocacy failed, her mother advised her to become "especially compliant" in order to gain her release. This 'compliance as the best strategy' is mirrored in the choices made by the other two women in their efforts to cope with the abuse.

Although this 'compliant' behavior may be interpreted as passive—and perhaps consensual to the officers seeking sex—the environmental context of a confined institutional setting must be considered. For example, similar to the situation illustrated by Fine (1984), Monica and Rhonda also made conscious decisions not to report the abuse because of the consequences such a disclosure might bring. In fact, their 'compliance' and seemingly strategic passivity reflect careful planning toward the greatest degree of safety—discharge from prison. Understanding the importance of context—and the women's long-term goal of getting out of the prison—we (re)classified their coping strategies. Using the original categories from the Ways of Coping (Folkman & Lazarus, 1980) instrument, we redefined behaviors, conceptualizing the possibilities within the setting and goal-oriented behavior to which the women ascribed. Thus, many behaviors that would traditionally be considered passive are translated as 'planful problem solving'—an active form of coping that has been found to be very efficacious (See Table 1).

TABLE 1 Coping Strategic Defined within the Environmental Context

Passive coping	Active coping
Distancing	Confrontive
(M) "I'm OK now"	(J) Attempted to file report
(M) "Yeah, right, whatever"	(J) Refused to comply with order
	to "inform" on others
(M) "Like I wasn't there"	(M) Kept journal
(M) Avoided talking about it	(R) Asked him to stop
	(R) Tried to quit work crew
Self controlling	Seeking social support
(M) Kept herself from fighting	(J) Used social network/family
Accepting Responsibility	(M) Told therapist
(M) Did not say no	(ALL 3) Involvement in lawsuit
Escape-avoidance	Planful problem solving/accommodative
(J) Walked away from harasser	(J) Did her "extra duty" to avoid conflict
and did not say anything	and get out on time
(J) Overeating	(M) Followed order to have sex to avoid write-up
(M) Wanted to be dead	(M) Did not want to report or prosecute to
(M) Withdrawn, irritable	avoid retaliation
(M) "Was going to kill myself"	(M) Kept condom from officer for fear of
(M) Attempted suicide	retaliation ticket
	(M) Kept condoms on desk to be found
	in shakedown
	(M) Did not resist again for fear of new case,
	segregation
	(M) Overdosed on Haldol to get to hospital
	– away from prison
	(R) Did not file grievance because she wanted
	to be released
	(R) Complied to avoid receiving an escape ticket
	(R) Refused meds because it would delay parole
Positive reappraisal	
(J) Felt she grew up a lot	
as a result	
(M) "Didn't think I'd be as	
strong as I am now"	

Note. M = Monica (Case 1); R = Rhonda (Case 2): J = June (Case 3).

Literature on coping has traditionally categorized emotion-focused coping as a feminine strategy that is less efficacious than problem-focused coping, which is associated with males (Banyard & Graham-Bermann, 1993). In fact, Western cultural norms devalue and stigmatize individuals who utilize avoidant or emotion-focused coping strategies, which are commonly practiced by abuse survivors (Morrow & Smith, 1995). Our goal, similar to that of Compas and colleagues (2001), is to transcend the dualistic framework of "passive/disengaged" and "active/engaged," which inherently implies "bad" and "good" solutions. It is our intention to expand upon current understandings of coping by including the factors of the individual's appraisal of the stressful event and the environment in which it occurs. By drawing upon the cognitive–transactional framework, we assess the reciprocal relationship between individual and environment (Lazarus & Folkman, 1984) leading to perhaps a third category. This third category, accommodation, has been described as coping efforts that adapt to the situation "through cognitive methods of reframing, acceptance, or distraction" (Compas et al., 2001).

A history of sexual abuse seriously impacts the appraisal process to the degree that one's perception of one's personal resources is limited. Children who are sexually abused seldom use problem-focused coping because they do not anticipate positive outcomes (Long & Jackson, 1993; Morrow & Smith, 1995). Similarly, incarcerated women who are sexually abused—and may enter prison with histories of childhood sexual assault—understand that problem-focused coping may be impossible or ineffective because they cannot remove themselves from the current situation. The extreme power differentials that exist in prison require coping that sustains survival—perhaps sacrificing short-term action, which may result in more harm, for long-term safety.

The women involved in this class action suit ultimately decided to do something other than accommodate the abuse. Their collective involvement in a lawsuit against the DOC represents a very active and, some may argue, risky coping strategy. Many of the women were still inside the prison when the lawsuit began and were subjected to further retaliation by staff. Although they won the lawsuit with monetary damages and promised reforms, the changes have been slow to come and a new lawsuit involving hundreds of other women is underway. This type of problem/solution-focused strategy may not be available to all women experiencing prison or jail abuse. In this particular location, a very committed group of attorneys has worked with the women for over twenty years on various reforms. This long-term alliance facilitated a trusting relationship that eventually enabled women to share their abuse stories with the attorneys.

Practitioners need to be aware of the circumstances that women face during incarceration and be prepared to offer multi-level interventions. These interventions must target the individual, system, and policy levels—simultaneously anticipating the needs of women during their incarceration and upon community re-entry, while eliminating the abusive institutional environment. Interventions at the individual level include efforts to empower women and facilitate meaningful connections. Incarceration clearly restricts control of the environment, but the Peer Support Team model suggested by Heney and Kristiansen (1997) is one example of self-empowerment that can be useful in enhancing a sense of efficacy within the institution. Trained teams of incarcerated women provide women-centered support and crisis intervention to their peers. Similar models may be helpful to women as they re-enter the community because the shame associated with such prison-based abuse may be too painful to share with others who may or may not believe them or understand why they made certain choices.

Practitioners within these facilities must make efforts to establish therapeutic alliances with incarcerated women in order to provide them with opportunities to build trust and confidence. However, before such alliances are made, each clinician must wrestle with the ethical dilemmas inherent within the position he or she holds. The challenge for clinicians is to navigate the complex demands of client advocacy and employer (e.g., DOC) expectations and policies.

Practitioners must be aware of other symptoms of psychological distress associated with trauma. Although, as indicated previously, our goal was to investigate conscious efforts to reduce stress (coping), it is important to acknowledge the use of dissociation (i.e., disruption in the usually integrated functions of consciousness), as an unconscious strategy to reduce anxiety. This defense mechanism, illustrated in Monica's case narrative, should be recognized as a response common to abuse survivors and to those with PTSD.

Many women may benefit from the use of psychopharmacological treatments to deal with the symptoms of depression and/or anxiety secondary to the current or past abuse. These treatments should be available without negative repercussions for parole—and thus may become one targeted intervention that requires attention at the individual, system, and policy levels.

At the institutional and policy levels, practitioners need to advocate for policies that are consistent with international human-rights standards (see Geer, 2000). Based on those standards, we recommend the complete elimination of male guards from female housing units. In addition, we advocate for specific education and training of staff on the sequalae associated with abuse and trauma exposure.

Furthermore, in order to establish a continuum of care and decrease the incidence of recidivism and relapse, planning for reintegration must begin as women enter the prison system (Wilson & Anderson, 1997). Richie (2001) found that neighborhood conditions, community resources, and public policies, as well as access to services for mental-health and substance-abuse treatment, housing, and employment, had a profound impact on women's reentry into their communities. Specifically, substance use as a coping strategy must be recognized prior to discharge and addressed with treatment strategies that are efficacious but realistic as well, given the unique circumstances of incarcerated women. We recommend that these areas be addressed at multiple levels.

Recently the Prison Rape Reduction Act was signed by President Bush to address the problem and decrease its frequency through more vigilant monitoring. Interestingly, the legislation solely refers to prisoner-on-prisoner rape, a phenomenon more common in male institutions, and fails to address staff-on-inmate rape. This omission perpetuates the systemic oppression of women within the criminal justice system by repeating the historical trend of creating and sustaining policies based on the needs of males, while ignoring those specific to women. This forgotten group of women deserves a voice in policy-making in order to create settings that are appropriate for their needs—those which offer healing, empowerment, and self-efficacy in a safe environment that is void of sexual assault. As Monica reminds us, "I came to prison to do my time—not to get raped."

NOTES

1. Among these reasons is protection of the women who may share information and continue to be subjected to incarceration. Therefore, we could not in good conscience complete a Human Subjects Investigation Committee application knowing that we could not protect the women who participated in such a study.

2. Names have been changed to protect anonymity.

REFERENCES

Amnesty International. (1999). *"Not part of my sentence": Violations of the human rights of women in custody.* London: Author.

Banyard, V. L. and Graham-Bermann, S. A. (1993). Can women cope? A gender analysis of theories of coping with stress. *Psychology of Women Quarterly, 17,* 303–318.

Beck, A. (2000). *Prison and jail inmates at midyear 1999* (NCJ Publication No.181643). Washington, DC: US Department of Justice, Office of Justice Programs.

Brandell, J. and Vargas, T. (2001). Narrative Case Studies. In B. Thyer (Ed.), *The Handbook of Social Work Research Methods* (pp. 293–307). Thousand Oaks, CA: Sage Publications.

Breslau, N., Davis, G. C., Peterson, E. L., and Schultz, L. (1997). Psychiatric sequelae of posttraumatic stress disorder in women. *Archives of General Psychiatry, 54*(1), 81–88.

Bureau of Justice Statistics. (1994). *Women in prison* (NCJ Publication No. 145321). Washington, DC: Author.

Compas, B. E., Connor-Smith, J. K., Saltzman, H., Thomsen, A. H., and Wadsworth, M. E. (2001). Coping with stress during childhood and adolescence: Problems, progress, and potential in theory and research. *Psychological Bulletin, 127,* 87–127.

Cottler, L. B., Compton, W. M., Mager, D., Spitznagel, E. L., and Janca, A. (1992). Posttraumatic stress disorder among substance abusers from the general population. *The American Journal of Psychiatry, 149*(5), 664–670.

Dansky, B. S., Brady, K. T., and Saladin, M. E. (1998). Untreated symptoms of PTSD among cocaine dependent individuals: Changes over time. *Journal of Substance Abuse Treatment, 15*(6), 499–504.

Fine, M. (1984). Coping with rape: Critical perspectives on consciousness. *Imagination, Cognition, and Personality, 3,* 249–267.

Folkman, S. and Lazarus, R. (1980). An analysis of coping in a middle-aged community sample. *Journal of Health and Social Behavior, 21,* 219–239.

Folkman, S. and Lazarus, R. (1985). If it changes it must be a process: Study of emotion and coping during three stages of a college examination. *Journal of Personality and Social Psychology, 48*(1), 150–170.

Freyd, J. J. (1996). *Betrayal Trauma.* Cambridge, MA: Harvard University Press.

Geer, M. (2000). Human rights and wrongs in our own backyard: Incorporating international human rights protections under domestic civil rights law – A case study of women in U. S. prisons. *Harvard Human Rights Journal, 13,* 71–140.

Gilgun, J. (2001). Case research designs. In R. M. Grinnell (Ed.), *Social work research and evaluation: Quantitative and qualitative approaches* (6th Ed.) (pp. 260–273). Itasca, IL: F.E. Peacock Publishers.

Greenfeld, L. and Snell, T. (1999). *Women offenders: Bureau of Justice Statistics special report* (NCJ Publication No. 175688). Washington, DC: U.S. Department of Justice.

Hearn, J. and Parkin, W. (2001). *Gender, sexuality and violence in organizations: The unspoken forces of organizational violence.* London: Sage Publications.

Heney, J. and Kristiansen, C. (1997). An analysis of the impact of prison on women survivors of childhood sexual abuse. *Women & Therapy, 20*(4), 29–44.

Herman, J. L. (1992). *Trauma and Recovery.* New York: Basic Books.

Human Rights Watch. (1996). *All too familiar: Sexual abuse of women in U.S. state prisons.* New York: Author.

Jordan, B. K., Schlenger, W. E., Fairbank, J. A., and Caddell, J. M. (1996). Prevalence of psychiatric disorders among incarcerated women. *Archives of General Psychiatry, 53,* 513–519.

Kaiser, C. R. and Miller, C. T. (2004). A stress and coping perspective on confronting sexism. *Psychology of Women Quarterly, 28,* 168–178.

Krysik, J. (2001). Secondary analysis. In R. M. Grinnell (Ed.), *Social work research and evaluation: Quantitative and qualitative approaches* (6th Ed.) (pp. 260–273). Itasca, IL; F.E. Peacock Publishers.

Kubiak, S. P. (in press). The primary and secondary effects of assault and harassment of women during incarceration.

Kubiak, S. P., Boyd, C., Slayden, J., and Young, A. (in press). Assessment of the substance abuse treatment needs of prisoners: Implementation of an integrated statewide approach. *Journal of Offender Rehabilitation.*

Kubiak, S. P., Siefert, K., and Boyd, C. (2004). Empowerment and public policy: An exploration of the implications of Section 115 of the Personal Responsibility and Work Opportunity Act. *Journal of Community Psychology, 32*(2), 127–143.

LaBelle, D. (2002). Women, the law, and the justice system: Neglect, violence, and resistance. In J. Figueira and R. C. Sarri (Eds.), *Women at the margins: Neglect, punishment, and resistance* (pp. 347–369). New York: Haworth Press.

LaBelle, D. and Kubiak, S. P. (2004). Baloncing gender equity for women prisoners. *Feminist Studies, 30*, 416–426.

Landrine, H. and Klonoff, E. A. (1996). The schedule of racist events: A measure of racial discrimination and a study of negative physical and mental health consequences. *Journal of Black Psychology, 22*(2), 144–156.

Lazarus, R. S. and Folkman, S. (1984). *Stress appraisal and coping.* New York: Springer Publications.

Long, P. J. and Jockson, J. L. (1993). Childhood coping strategies and the adult adjustment of female sexual abuse victims. *Journal of Child Sexual Abuse, 2*(2), 23–29.

Lykes, M. (1983). Discrimination and coping in the lives of black women: Analyses of oral history data. *Journal of Social Issues, 39*(3), 79–100.

Mauer, M., Potler, C., and Wolf, R. (1999). *Gender and justice: Women, drugs, and sentencing policy.* Washington, DC: The Sentencing Project.

Morash, M., Bynum, T. S., and Koons, B. A. (1998). *Women offenders: Programming needs and promising approaches.* Washington, DC: U.S. Department of Justice, National Institute of Justice.

Morash, M. and Schram, P. J. (2002). *The prison experience: Special issues of women in prison.* Prospect Heights, IL: Waveland Press.

Morrow, S. L. and Smith, M. L. (1995). Constrictions of survival and coping by women who have survived childhood sexual abuse. *Journal of Counseling Psychology, 42*(1), 24–33.

National Institute of Justice. (April 2003). 2000 Arrestee Drug Abuse Monitoring.

Pearlin, L., Menaghan, E., and Lieberman, M. (1981). The stress process. *Journal of Health and Social Behavior, 22*, 337–356.

Pimlott, S. and Sarri, R. (2002). The forgotten group: Women in prisons and jails. In R. Sarri and J. Figueira-McDonough (Eds.), *Women at the margins: Surviving neglect and punishment.* Binghamton, NY: Hayworth Press.

Riessman, C. K. (2001). Analysis of personal narratives. In J. F. Gubrium and J. A. Holstein (Eds.), *Handbook of Interviewing*, Sage Publications.

Richie, B. E. (2001). Challenges incarcerated women face as they return to their communities: Findings from life history interviews. *Crime and Delinquency, 47*(3), 368–389.

Smith, C. A. and Lazarus, R. A. (1989). Emotion and adaptation. In L. A. Pervin & O. P. John (Eds.), *Handbook of personality* (1st Ed.) (pp. 609–637). New York: Guilford Press.

Stewart, S., Ouimette, P., and Brown, P. J. (2003). Gender and the comorbidity of PTSD with substance use disorders. In R. Kimmerling, P. Ouimettem, & J. Wolfe (Eds.), *Gender and PTSD.* New York: Guilford Press.

Teplin, L. A., Abram, K. M., and McClelland, G. M. (1996). The prevalence of psychiatric disorder among incarcerated women, I: Pre-trial jail detainees. *Archives of General Psychiatry, 53*, 505–512.

U.S. General Accounting Office. (1999). *Women in prison: Sexual misconduct by correctional staff* (Report No. GAO/GGD-99-104). Washington, DC: Author.

Wilson, M. K. and Anderson, S. C. (1997). Empowering female offenders: Removing barriers to community-based practice. *Affilia, 12*(3), 342–358.

7

Integrating Research and Practice: A Collaborative Model for Addressing Trauma and Addiction

SHELLY A. WIECHELT, WENDY LUTZ,
NANCY J. SMYTH, and CHARLES SYMS
*School of Social Work, University at Buffalo, State University of New York,
Buffalo, New York, USA*

Research findings on trauma and substance abuse have led researchers to conclude that trauma, especially childhood trauma, is an important risk factor for the development of substance use disorders (SUD; Cottler, Compton, Mager, Spitznagel, & Janca, 1992; Miller, Downs & Testa, 1993). Comorbidity research indicates that posttraumatic stress disorder (PTSD) and SUD co-occur at high rates (Kessler, Sonnega, Bromet, Hughes, & Nelson, 1995; Rosenberg et al., 2001; Stewart, 1996). Nevertheless, there is continuing debate on how the relationship between trauma and SUD operates. Some argue that PTSD causes the SUD while others suggest that SUD increases the risk for trauma and thus PTSD (Chilcoat & Breslau, 1998; Chilcoat & Menard, 2003; Stewart, Pihl, Conrod, & Dongier, 1998). It has also been suggested that once the disorder develops, the symptoms of one disorder maintain the symptoms of the other (Stewart, 1996). Although most agree that both the PTSD and SUD warrant treatment, there is debate on both the timing (sequential vs. integrated) and type of treatment (Najavits, 2003). In any case, it is essential that practitioners assess clients who abuse substances on their history of traumatic experiences and provide appropriate interventions or referrals to them. Even though it is clear that there are links between trauma and SUD, most addiction treatment programs do not provide assessment or treatment for trauma or PTSD. Consequently, addicted clients are often left with a significant component of their problem unaddressed. Failure to appropriately address the impact of clients' trauma histories has been cited as a factor that contributes to relapse (Brown, 2000; Evans & Sullivan, 1995).

To respond to these issues, a group of researchers and practitioners who were members of the Western New York Practice Research Network (WNY-PRN) developed an initiative to redress clinicians' reluctance to assess or provide interventions to address trauma in addiction-treatment settings. The collaborative group consisted of faculty from the University at Buffalo School of Social Work, directors from community agencies, and the Director of Dual Recovery Services from Erie County, New York. The purpose of the WNY-PRN is to promote collaboration between researchers and practitioners in an effort to encourage research based practice and practice informed research. The group developed an initiative that included resource development, training, and research. The project was conducted in two phases. Funding for each phase of the project was obtained via grants through the New York State Practice Improvement Collaborative. This paper reports on each phase of the project and the process of this unique collaboration between researchers and practitioners.

PHASE I

The aims of Phase I of the project were to: Identify and acquire trauma screening instruments that could be used within agency settings; obtain input from clinicians on the utility of the trauma screening instruments and their views on incorporating trauma screening interviews into assessments; identify and obtain evidenced-based and best-practice resources to be used to address the needs of addicted trauma survivors; and plan and implement trainings to educate staff about: (a) trauma and addiction, (b) use of the selected assessment instruments, and (c) availability of resources.

The planning group met monthly to address the project's aims. The group reviewed for purchase resource materials that addressed trauma and addiction, such as videos, treatment manuals, and books. The selected resources were purchased and placed in central county agencies where all clinicians could access them. A flyer describing the contents of the library was distributed to community agencies. Two training options were developed and offered. First, a member of the planning group provided the *Risking Connection* training (Saakvitne, Gamble, Pearlman & Lev, 2000) to clinicians at the agencies whose directors were participating in the project. Second, a three-day regional training on trauma and addiction was planned for implementation in Phase II of the project (described in detail later in this paper.) The regional training was offered to any interested practitioner through the Continuing Education Program at the University at Buffalo School of Social Work. The planning group also identified trauma screening tools that may be useful for clinicians in addiction treatment settings and obtained data on the clinicians' views of these instruments in particular and on trauma screening in general in two focus groups. The methods that were used for the focus groups and the results from them are reported below.

Method

PARTICIPANTS

Clinicians from inpatient and outpatient addiction-treatment programs in the vicinity of Buffalo, New York, were recruited via telephone calls and e-mails sent to agency directors. Directors were asked to identify two volunteers from their staff (one clinical supervisor and one member of the line staff) who would be willing to participate in a focus group examining trauma-screening instruments for use in the assessment process. Two focus groups were held. The first group consisted of eight inpatient staff; five of the inpatient participants were line staff and three were supervisors. The staff represented five agencies. The second group consisted of nine staff members from outpatient substance abuse treatment programs; six of the outpatient participants were line staff and three were supervisors. Six outpatient programs were represented.

MEASURES

The planning group identified three measures that were designed to assess individuals on their experience of potentially traumatic events: The Parent-Child Conflict Tactics Scales (PCCTS; Straus, Hamby, Finkelhor, & Runyan, 1995), the National Women's Study–PTSD Module–Part I (NWS–PI;

Kilpatrick, Resnick, Saunders, & Best, 1989), and the Violence and Trauma Screening Questionnaire for Human Service Agencies (VTSQ; District of Columbia Trauma Collaboration Study, 1999). Measure selection was based on ease of use, relevant content, and psychometric properties. The planning group determined that both the NWS—PI and the PCCTS had too much detail and were too long for clinicians to use as a screening tool during initial assessments. Consequently, the NWS-PI and the PCCTS were modified before being presented to the focus groups.

The original NWS-PI consists of 18 questions that ask whether an individual has experienced a certain traumatic event. The items cover the range of events that would be considered when determining if an individual meets DSM-IV Criterion A for a diagnosis of PTSD (see American Psychiatric Association, 1994). For each event that an individual affirms experiencing he or she is asked the following questions: his or her age at the time of the event; the description of the event; if perpetrated by another, who was the perpetrator; and if the respondent thought he or she would die or be injured during the event. Individuals are probed for all incidents of each type of event. A sample item is "Has anyone ever made you have anal sex by using force or threatening to harm you or someone close to you? Just so there is no mistake, by anal sex we mean a man or boy putting his penis in your anus." Resnick (1996) notes that there are highly comparable rates of specific and multiple event exposure between the NWS-PI and other measures of traumatic events across general population studies, thus supporting its validity.

The modified version of the NWS-PI that was evaluated in the focus groups included all 18 of the items from the original NWS-PI. The follow-up probe questions were modified. Data were to be gathered on the age of the client and the perpetrator's identity for the first event only. If additional incidents of the event were reported to have occurred, it would be noted only under the number of events. No additional details were to be gathered.

The NWS-PTSD Module has a second part that can be used in tandem with Part I to determine if an individual meets criteria for a diagnosis of post-traumatic stress disorder (PTSD). Part II was not used in this study as the intent was to identify a useful screening tool to determine if clients had traumatic experiences, rather than to determine if they were experiencing PTSD. For a discussion of the entire NWS-PTSD Module, see Resnick, Kilpatrick, Dansky, Saunders, and Best (1993).

PARENT-CHILD CONFLICT TACTICS SCALES

The PCCTS is comprised of three scales: 1) physical assault (minor assault, severe assault, and very severe assault), 2) psychological aggression, and

3) non-violent discipline. There are also three supplemental scales: 1) weekly discipline, 2) neglect, and 3) sexual abuse. The total possible number of items when the supplement scales are included is 35. The items can be formatted to ask parents about their behavior toward their children, children about the behavior of their parents, and adults about their parents' behavior towards them when they were children. Like its predecessor, the Conflict Tactics Scale (Straus, Hamby, McCoy, & Sugarman, 1996), the PCCTS has low internal-consistency reliability. The authors suggest that this is due to the fact that the items measure rare events, resulting in a skewed distribution and lowered correlations (Straus, Hamby, Finkelhor, Moore, & Runyan, 1998). Straus, et al. (1998) present evidence to support that the PCCTS has construct validity.

The PCCTS that was evaluated in the focus groups was formatted for adult recall. Items from all but the weekly discipline scale were used to develop the modified version of the PCCTS that was used in the focus-group study. Since the intended use of the instrument in this project was to screen clients for traumatic experiences, several of the items were collapsed together. Also, the response categories for each item were changed from ranking the frequency of the occurrence to 'yes' and 'no' categories. Probes on the age the client was when the event occurred and who perpetrated the act were added to the measure. The modified PCCTS consisted of 15 items. A sample item from the modified PCCTS that was evaluated in the focus groups asked: "When you were a child or teenager did your parent(s) or guardian(s) shake, hit, kick, choke, slap, or punch you?"; if yes, "what age(s) did this happen and who did this to you?"

VIOLENCE AND TRAUMA SCREENING QUESTIONNAIRE FOR HUMAN
SERVICE AGENCIES (VTSQ)

The VTSQ is a measure that was created by a subcommittee of the District of Columbia Trauma Collaboration Study (District of Columbia Trauma Collaboration Study, 1999). The measure consists of eight items that were taken from various instruments and interviews on trauma. A sample item is: "At any time in your life have you witnessed a physical or sexual assault against a family member, friend, or significant person?" There are follow-up probes on the age the event happened and on whether the event occurred in the past 12 months. There is an extensive introduction to the measure that describes the experience of violence in general, ways people react to violence, and the nature of the questions that are about to be asked. The introduction is geared to women. The measure is intended to be used as a brief screening tool in human-service agencies. The psychometric properties of the measure have not been evaluated. The VTSQ was not revised for use in the focus groups for this study.

INTERVIEW GUIDE

An interview guide was developed for use in the focus groups. It consisted of five questions on the participants' views on screening for trauma during addiction treatment including benefits, problems, ways of resolving said problems, and what types of training and support clinicians would need to use trauma screening tools. Each of the three trauma screening tools selected by the planning group (NWS-PI, PCCTS, and VTSQ) was evaluated on the following four points: 1) The structure of the instrument, 2) its clinical utility, 3) the feasibility of using it within the clinical setting, and 4) its overall advantages and disadvantages. The trauma screening tools were also placed in rank order by the participants on the aforementioned categories.

PROCEDURES

The focus groups were held in a conference room at a local treatment center. Participants were seated around a conference table. Each participant was given a nametag and asked to sign in. Once all participants had arrived, the informed consent was reviewed with them. They were informed about the purpose and procedure of the focus group. The participants were told that their participation was voluntary and confidential and that the views discussed in the group would be reported anonymously. Discussion began after the informed consents were signed.

A researcher facilitated each focus group using the interview guide and a research assistant recorded comments on a flip chart. The groups were also audio-taped for the purpose of verifying comments only. The procedures were reviewed and approved by the Institutional Review Board of the University at Buffalo. The data obtained from each focus group were analyzed for themes and compared to the other focus group. Since responses were similar, the results from both focus groups are summarized together below.

Results

VIEWS ON TRAUMA SCREENING

BENEFITS OF TRAUMA SCREENING

Focus-group participants expressed that they believed that trauma is a major issue for addicted people. They indicated that they recognized that the effects of trauma influenced drinking and drug use and vice versa. Several ways of conducting trauma screening in the assessment process to benefit clients were identified. The participants indicated that the information gathered from the trauma screening would give counselors insight into the client's strengths, beliefs, behaviors, coping styles, and defensive strategies, thus, giving the counselor a better understanding of the client's treatment needs. Also, having information on the role that trauma has played in the addicted person's life would help the clinician to develop a holistic view of the client's problems. The participants also stated that the information obtained from trauma screening would help in the process of identifying which counselor would be most appropriate to work with the client. All of these factors would contribute to improved treatment for the clients.

CONCERNS ABOUT TRAUMA SCREENING

Focus-group participants expressed several concerns about the impact that assessing trauma would have on clients beginning substance-abuse treatment. They expressed that focusing too heavily on trauma in the assessment process would diminish the emotional safety of the client. It was suggested that trauma screening in the initial assessment may be "too much too soon." Participants indicated that the trauma assessment could overwhelm clients and potentially scare them away. They were concerned that asking clients about their exposure to trauma might trigger traumatic memories or symptoms. This would be particularly problematic for clients in outpatient settings who are often not seen for a week or more after the initial assessment. Clients who experienced an increase in traumatic memories and symptoms would be at increased risk for resuming substance use or not returning for treatment.

The focus-group participants identified potential problems with integrating the trauma screening into the initial assessment due to the limitations of the staff or agency. They pointed out that some staff and agencies held treatment philosophies that trauma should not be addressed too early in treatment. Further, that the staff may be afraid to ask about trauma issues. They were concerned that they, themselves, or other counselors that they worked with were not trained to conduct trauma screening or to handle the emotional and psychological upset that asking about trauma might provoke in their clients. This lack of training could result in the client being retraumatized by the interview. Focus-group participants reported that they were generally allotted $1-1\frac{1}{2}$ hours to conduct their assessment and were concerned that they did not have time to add more questions to their assessment. The participants were also concerned that if clients did become upset by the questions about trauma, there would not be enough time to sufficiently address the client's needs and finish the assessment interview.

STRATEGIES TO OVERCOME CONCERNS

The focus-group participants suggested the following strategies for overcoming the problems that might arise with conducting trauma screenings in their agencies:

- Staff should be trained on conducting trauma screenings and receive good supervision;
- Clinicians should be taught how to care for themselves when working with clients on trauma issues and how to avoid vicarious traumatization;

- Agencies should match clients with clinicians who are best able to meet their treatment needs;
- Treatment programs should provide gender-specific treatment groups, safe places in treatment, and additional support for those clients dealing with trauma in addition to substance abuse;
- The screening instrument should be brief and should be administered after trust and rapport have been established in the interview;
- More time should be allotted for the initial assessment;
- Procedures should be established to ensure that the treatment team receives information on the client's experience of trauma and appropriate supports, referrals, and interventions are provided to the client.

TRAINING AND SUPPORT

Focus-group participants identified the kinds of training or support that would be needed for staff to integrate trauma assessment into the initial assessment in their agencies. Training suggestions included the nature of trauma, types of trauma, symptoms and diagnosis of posttraumatic stress disorder (PTSD), links between trauma and substance abuse, assessing and screening for trauma, and treatment approaches to address trauma and addiction. It was also suggested that all treatment team members including doctors, nurses, social workers, psychologists, counselors, etc. receive training on trauma so that the team could act in unison.

SUMMARY OF VIEWS ON SCREENING TOOLS

PARENT CHILD CONFLICT TACTICS SCALE

Participants found this instrument to be too narrow and repetitive. They indicated that there was too much detail and that the questions were too specific for an initial assessment. It was suggested that this instrument might be too overwhelming and scare clients away from treatment. It was also pointed out that the PCCTS does not ask about catastrophic event trauma or post-teen trauma. Participants ranked the PCCTS third in all categories. The participants thought that the instrument could be useful as a guide to counselors on what questions to ask when they were assessing clients for trauma. It was suggested that the counselor would have to use his or her judgment on which questions to ask and how much detail should be gathered.

NATIONAL WOMEN'S SURVEY–PTSD MODULE, PART I

Focus-group participants ranked the NWS-PI second on all categories. They expressed that it was "softer" or more sensitive, and therefore better than the PCCTS. They thought that the introductory and connecting narratives were helpful. Also, the NWS-PI covers the range of potentially traumatic events that a person might experience. On the other hand, participants observed that the questions about sexual abuse were too intense, too detailed, and too specific for an initial interview. They stated that the specific sexual references in the questions might cause some discomfort for clinicians as well. It was suggested that the questions could be rank ordered and asked at different stages of the assessment.

Violence and Trauma Screening Questionnaire

Focus-group participants indicated that the VTSQ was the best of the three instruments. The instrument seemed to be non-threatening and client centered. They suggested that since the instrument is brief and does not ask for specific details, it is well suited for an initial assessment interview. The participants noted that the introduction to the VTSQ would be helpful in preparing the client for the questions, but would need to be reworded to be gender neutral. Additionally, the VTSQ seemed to be more empowering than the other two instruments, specifically in that it gives clients the option of stopping the interview. One concern was that the VTSQ asks about past and current traumatic events, but does not ask about catastrophic events or war trauma.

Discussion

In sum, participants expressed a belief that trauma should be assessed during the initial assessment of addiction problems. The initial assessment of trauma should be a brief screening that should be followed up with a more in-depth trauma assessment by the primary counselor. Participants were concerned that even a screening interview may be overwhelming for clients and that staff should be trained to conduct the screening and handle trauma issues. Also, staff should be allotted more time to conduct assessments. They suggested that agency policy be established on how to handle clients who become upset when trauma issues are screened for or addressed. Focus-group participants ranked the VTSQ first in terms of (a) instrument structure, (b) clinical utility, (c) feasibility of use in an assessment setting, and (d) overall impression. They ranked the NWS-PI second and the PCCTS third in all of the above categories. The participants also indicated that the VTSQ would provide them with the information needed on the client's experience of trauma while being minimally intrusive.

The findings from the focus groups indicate that the clinicians generally believed that trauma is an issue for the clients with whom they work and that screening is helpful. The clinicians were concerned that either they or the agency lacked the resources to address trauma once it is exposed. Many practitioners felt they lacked specific training on trauma. They felt uncomfortable asking about trauma and did not know how to proceed when a trauma history is identified in their clients. It appears that it would be beneficial if agencies would provide training and support to their staff members on assessing trauma and making appropriate referrals or providing interventions. Agencies need to make structural changes in their programs to allow trauma issues to be assessed or addressed. For example, more time could be allotted for completing assessments, certain staff could be trained in trauma issues and assigned clients for individual or group work on their trauma issues, and programs could be restructured to systematically address the frequently comorbid PTSD and SUD disorders.

PHASE II

Phase II of the project was a pilot study on the two instruments that were most highly ranked in the focus groups (VTSQ and NWS-PI). The specific aim of the pilot study was to identify which screening tool is most useful to clinicians in actual practice settings. The planning group met bimonthly to plan, monitor, and discuss the pilot study.

Method

PARTICIPANTS

Clinicians from five Western New York substance-abuse treatment facilities (two inpatient facilities and three outpatient facilities) participated in the pilot study. The directors of these treatment programs were members of this project's planning group and volunteered their agencies to participate in the pilot test. The data on the clinicians' views on each instrument were gathered at staff meetings. Not all staff who used the instruments were present at every meeting. A total of 27 clinicians completed the survey on NWS-PI and 21 clinicians completed the survey on the VTSQ.

MEASURES

The NWS-PI and VTSQ were revised to incorporate suggestions that were made by the participants in the focus groups. The NWS-PI was shortened by combining items that were similar. For example, rather than asking four questions on different types of forced sex, all of the forced-sex items were combined into one item: "Has someone ever made you have sex by using force, threatening to harm you or someone close to you? By sex we mean fingers or objects in your vagina or anus, and oral and anal sex." The introduction to the VTSQ was revised to make it gender-neutral. These two measures were used by the clinicians in their initial assessment of clients.

A measure of the clinicians' views on each trauma screening tool was developed by the planning group. It consisted of nine items on a five-point scale with lower scores indicating a high level of agreement and higher scores indicating a low level of agreement. A sample item was, "The instrument is easy to use." Participants were also asked to list the advantages and disadvantages of each instrument.

PROCEDURES

Clinicians were informed that their treatment programs were participating in the pilot project and were instructed to incorporate the trauma screening instruments into their assessment by the directors of their programs. A research assistant went to a staff meeting at each participating agency and distributed the NWS-PI and explained how it should be used. After the four-week NWS-PI trial was completed, the research assistant returned to each agency and administered the questionnaire on the clinicians' views of the instrument. The clinicians were informed that their participation in filling out the questionnaire was completely voluntary and confidential. There was no identifying information on the questionnaire, thus the clinicians' responses were anonymous. Participating clinicians did sign an informed consent. The VTSQ was distributed and explained during a staff meeting at each participating treatment program. At the end of the four-week VTSQ trial, the research assistant returned to each program's staff meeting and, using the procedures described above, administered the questionnaire on clinicians' attitudes towards the instrument. The procedures used in the pilot study were reviewed and approved by the Institutional Review Board at the University at Buffalo.

Results

The clinicians' views on the two measures were compared using t-tests. There was no significant difference between the NWS-PI and the VTSQ when total mean scores were compared. The total mean scores were 2.4 (.60) and 2.2 (.48), respectively, indicating that the clinicians had positive attitudes towards both trauma screening instruments. Table 1 shows item-by-item comparisons on the clinicians views of the trauma screening tools and reveals that the clinicians viewed the VTSQ as being better designed and easier to use than the NWS-PI.

The participants' comments on the surveys indicated a preference for the VTSQ. Comments on the NWS-PI evaluation included: "The design was cumbersome"; "Difficult to follow"; "This was hard to do during an assessment...it is a bit overwhelming [for clients]"; "This gave a more in-depth view of the client's issues"; "Actually found out more incidents of trauma"; and "Easy for client to understand." Comments on the VTSQ evaluation included: "Quick to complete"; "Time effective"; "Serves as an introduction to further exploration"; "Info [*sic*] gathered was straightforward and

TABLE 1 Comparisons of Clinicians' Views on Trauma Screening Instruments

Item	NWS-PI $n = 27$	VTSQ $n = 21$	t
Well designed	2.70 (.91)	2.19 (.81)	2.03*
Easy to use	2.41 (.88)	1.90 (.83)	2.00*
Elicits useful information	2.00 (.83)	2.10 (.54)	−.46
Enhances overall assessment	2.30 (.72)	2.43 (.68)	−.65
Information will be useful in addressing client problems	2.15 (.77)	2.14 (.73)	.02
Realistic to use in a clinical setting	2.07 (.73)	1.90 (.63)	.85
Fits well into the assessment process	2.48 (.80)	2.62 (.81)	−.59
Can be incorporated into time frame of the assessment	2.63 (.97)	2.19 (.81)	1.67
Interferes with the assessment	2.44 (1.0)	2.48 (.75)	−.12

Note: Numbers in parentheses are standard deviations. t-tests all on 46 df.
*$p \leq .05$.

instrument was not intrusive"; and "Hard to fit this into initial psycho-social assessment." Although most comments on the evaluation of the NWS-PI included some disadvantages, only six of the evaluations on the VTSQ included disadvantages and most were about gathering information that was already gathered in one agency's standard evaluation.

Discussion

The findings from the pilot study suggest that the clinicians found both the VTSQ and the NWS-PI to be useful in clinical settings. They indicated that the VTSQ was easier to use and better designed than the NWS-PI. Their comments on the advantages and disadvantages of the instruments suggest a preference for the VTSQ.

The external validity of this study is limited by the study being conducted in a single geographic region with a small sample of clinicians. The attitudes and perceptions reported by the clinicians may be peculiar to them or the region that they are from. The measures that were used in the study were adapted and do not have established psychometric properties. Future research on the reliability and validity of the instruments would be helpful. Also, research on how screening for trauma in addiction treatment influences outcomes would help to support the need for agencies to make the necessary structural changes and invest in staff training.

PROCESS EVALUATION

The planning group met to discuss the process of their collaboration and its effects. A summary of the group's discussion is presented here. The agency managers reported that they learned that it is important to prepare staff for the introduction of a new agency practice or research project several months in advance in order to develop the staff's commitment to and ownership of the project. The managers indicated that it is important to follow-up with staff to insure that the new screenings are incorporated into day-to-day agency practice. Members of the group reported that participating in the research/ practice collaboration was useful because it allowed researchers to learn about the community and the needs of the practitioners and it allowed practitioners to learn about existing research on trauma as well as research methods. Some members are working together on other research projects as a result of the mutual relationships that they built by participating in the WNY-PRN. The planning group will work to encourage other researchers and practitioners to join the group and extend the group's collaborative efforts.

The planning group believes that the keys for a successful collaboration between researchers and practitioners are to (a) educate one another on the demands of each respective enterprise, (b) respect the expertise that each member brings, (c) engage in a mutual exchange of ideas, and (d) be aware that certain times of the month or year place higher demands on agency or university personnel, such as reviews, grading, and grant deadlines.

CONCLUSION

Even though an abundance of existing research indicates that there are links between trauma and substance-abuse, many substance-abuse treatment programs do not screen their clients for trauma experiences or provide them with treatment or referrals for trauma treatment (Kessler et al., 1995; Rosenberg et al., 2001; Stewart, 1996). The findings from the focus groups suggest that clinicians who work in substance-abuse treatment settings do recognize that trauma is often an issue for their clients that needs to be addressed. The clinicians seem to be concerned that asking questions about trauma in an initial interview may overwhelm the client and that they will not have the time or expertise to help the client manage the upset. The findings from the focus groups and the pilot study also suggest that clinicians have a preference for screening tools that are brief and don't ask for much specific detail on the traumatic experiences. It appears that clinicians who work in substance-abuse treatment settings may be more likely to complete trauma screening assessments with their clients when they have been provided with brief screening instruments, appropriate training, and clear support and guidelines for handling trauma from their agency and supervisors. Additional research with a larger and more representative sample of clinicians is needed to determine if and how these factors influence clinicians' willingness and ability to assess clients for traumatic experiences and associated problems.

This project seems to have contributed to both the overall process goal of creating a partnership between researchers and practitioners and the specific aims of identifying and providing resources and tools to clinicians that would enable them to conduct trauma screening. Researchers and practitioners can use this type of innovative collaboration in their communities to enhance and inform research and practice. Such collaborative groups can be used to develop treatment initiatives with the investment of stakeholders from the research and practice arenas.

ACKNOWLEDGEMENTS

This study was funded by the New York State Practice Improvement Collaborative. The authors would like to acknowledge the contributions that the members of the Western New York Practice Research Network made to this project.

REFERENCES

American Psychiatric Association (1994). *Diagnostic and statistical manual of mental disorders* (4th ed.). Washington, DC: Author.

Brown, P. J. (2000). Outcome in female patients with both substance use and posttraumatic stress disorders. *Alcoholism Treatment Quarterly, 18*(3), 127–135.

Chilcoat, H. D. and Breslau, N. (1998). Investigations of causal pathways between PTSD and drug use disorders. *Addictive Behaviors, 23*(6), 827–840.

Chilcoat, H. D. and Menard, C. (2003). Epidemiological investigations: Comorbidity of posttraumatic stress disorder and substance use disorder. In P. C. Ouimette & P. J. Brown (Eds.), *Trauma and substance abuse: Causes, consequences, and treatment of comorbid disorders.* Washington, DC: American Psychological Association.

Cottler, L. B., Compton, W. M., Mager, D., Spitznagel, E. L., and Janca, A. (1992). Posttraumatic stress disorder among substance users from the general population. *American Journal of Psychiatry, 149*(5), 664–670.

District of Columbia Trauma Collaboration Study (DCTCS) – Screening Subcommittee (1999). *Violence and Trauma Screening Questionnaire.* Unpublished instrument.

Evans, K. and Sullivan, J. M. (1995). *Treating the addicted survivor of trauma.* New York: Guilford.

Kessler, R. C., Sonnega, A., Bromet, E., Hughes, M., and Nelson, C. (1995). Posttraumatic stress disorder in the national comorbidity survey. *Archives of General Psychiatry, 52*(12), 1048–1060.

Kilpatrick, D. G., Resnick, H. S., Saunders, B. E., and Best, C. L. (1989). *The National Women's Study PTSD Module*. Unpublished instrument. Charleston, SC: National Crime Victims Research and Treatment Center, Department of Psychiatry and Behavioral Sciences, Medical University of South Carolina.

Miller, B. A., Downs, W. R., and Testa, M. (1993). Interrelationships between victimization experiences and women's alcohol use. *Journal of Studies on Alcohol*, Suppl. 11, 109–117.

Najavits, L. M. (2003). Seeking safety: A new psychotherapy for posttraumatic stress disorder and substance use disorder. In P. Quimette & P. J. Brown (Eds.), *Trauma and substance abuse: Causes, consequences, and treatment of comorbid disorders* (pp. 147–169). Washington, DC: American Psychological Association.

Resnick, H. (1996). Psychometric review of National Women's Study (NWS) Event History-PTSD Module. In B. H. Stamm (Ed.), *Measurement of stress, trauma, and adaptation*. Lutherville, MD: Sidran Press.

Resnick, H. S., Kilpatrick, D. G., Dansky, B. S., Saunders, B. E., and Best, C. L. (1993). Prevalence of civilian trauma and posttraumatic stress disorder in a representative national sample of women. *Journal of Consulting and Clinical Psychology*, *61*(6), 984–991.

Rosenberg, S. D., Mueser, K. T., Friedman, M. J., Gorman, P. G., Drake, R. E., Vidaver, R. M., et al. (2001). Developing effective treatments for posttraumatic disorders among people with severe mental illness. *Psychiatric Services*, *52*(11), 1453–1461.

Saakvitne, K. W., Gamble, S., Pearlman, L. A., and Lev, B. T. (2000). *Risking connection: A training curriculum for working with survivors of childhood abuse*. Lutherville, MD: Sidran Press.

Straus, M. A., Hamby, S. L., Finkelhor, D., Moore, D. W., and Runyan, D. (1998). Identification of child maltreatment with the Parent-Child Conflict Tactics Scales: Development and psychometric data from a national sample of American parents. *Child Abuse & Neglect, 22*(4), 249–270.

Straus, M. A., Hamby, S. L., Finkelhor, D., and Runyan, D. (1995). *The Parent-Child Conflict Tactics Scales: Form A*. Durham, NH: Family Research Laboratory, University of New Hampshire.

Straus, M. A., Hamby, S. L., McCoy, S., and Sugarman, D. B. (1996). The Revised Conflict Tactics Scales. *Journal of Family Issues, 17*(3), 283–316.

Stewart, S. H. (1996). Alcohol abuse in individuals exposed to trauma: A critical review. *Psychological Bulletin, 120*(1), 83–112.

Stewart, S. H., Pihl, R. O., Conrod, P. J., and Dongier, M. (1998). Functional associations among trauma, PTSD, and substance-related disorders. *Addictive Behaviors, 23*(6), 797–812.

8

Subthreshold PTSD: A Comparison of Alcohol, Depression, and Health Problems in Canadian Peacekeepers with Different Levels of Traumatic Stress

JEFFREY S. YARVIS, PATRICK S. BORDNICK, and
CHRISTINA A. SPIVEY

University of Georgia, Athens, GA, USA

DAVID PEDLAR

Veterans Affairs Canada, Charlottetown, Prince Edward Island, Canada

Posttraumatic stress disorder (PTSD) was initially introduced to the *Diagnostic and Statistical Manual*, 3rd edition (DSM-III; American Psychiatric Association, 1980) to describe the range of syndromal reactions to traumatic stressors. This range of reactions was built upon the categorical model of psychiatric disorders. In the quarter of a century since the publication of DSM-III, numerous studies have shown that the current diagnostic threshold established by the categorical model is valid across traumatized populations such as combat and peacekeeping veterans; victims of crime and sexual assault; victims of man-made and natural disasters; victims of motor vehicle accidents; and victims of political oppression. Moreover, PTSD does not appear to be a rare phenomenon. In PILOTS database alone, there are hundreds of empirical investigations reporting that rates of PTSD in non-clinical samples and the general population are much higher than reported before 2001. The resultant effect of these findings, coupled with the global war on terrorism, has been increased professional and public understanding of the pervasiveness of PTSD. Given the current awareness and attention to PTSD, forthcoming questions about early intervention for the disorder raised questions about the PTSD diagnosis and the clinical relevance of subthreshold variants.

There is, however, a scarcity of empirical research examining the taxonomic issues of posttraumatic stress disorder and its sub-clinical forms, and whether or not subthreshold mental health disorders should be used as indicators of looming health problems. The goal of this study was to compare groups of respondents with full PTSD, subthreshold PTSD, or no PTSD on indicators of impairment often associated with PTSD. In order to meet this goal the following questions were addressed:

- Will groups of peacekeepers with full, subthreshold or no PTSD score differently when compared on measures of alcohol (AUDIT), depressive symptoms (CES-D), and number of physical health problems (health questionnaire)?
- More specifically, will peacekeepers with full and subthreshold PTSD show statistically significant mean differences from the no PTSD group when compared on these measures?

This study represents the first step in determining the clinical relevance of subthreshold PTSD by asking if subthreshold groups differ statistically from groups with full PTSD or no PTSD. Groups of peacekeepers with full, subthreshold and no PTSD were compared on measures of alcohol use disorders, depression and physical health problems. Since the taxometrics of PTSD and subthreshold PTSD have been changed over time, one of the primary aims of this investigation was to conduct an extensive review of the taxonomic history of full and subthreshold PTSD in order to establish an empirically supported operational definition of subthreshold PTSD.

Current data suggest that approximately 10% of armed forces personnel deployed for combat, peacekeeping, or humanitarian disaster relief present with PTSD following their tour of duty (Schlenger, Fairbank, Jordan, & Caddell, 1999). Additionally, a considerable proportion (i.e., 10–25%) of those not meeting threshold diagnostic criteria for PTSD experience significant subsyndromal symptoms (Asmundson et al., in press; Schlenger et al., 1999). These statistics are not surprising given the multiple stressors and potentially threatening situations to which deployed military personnel are exposed.

An abundance of previous investigations document the association between PTSD symptoms and poor health in military veterans and others (for reviews see Resnick Acierno, & Kilpatrick, 1997; Schnurr & Jankowski, 1999). PTSD symptoms are associated with greater reporting of physical health problems and physical symptoms (Beckham et al., 1998; Kimerling, Clum, & Wolfe, 2000; Wagner, Wolfe, & Rotnitsky, 2000; Zatzick, Marmar, & Weiss, 1997). They are also strongly associated with psychological impairment, current pain and pain-related disability (Beckham et al., 1997), poorer functional outcomes (Kimerling et al., 2000; Wagner et al., 2000), and increased healthcare consumption (Marshall, Jorm, & Grayson, 1998). These findings appear to hold irrespective of deployment theater (e.g., Vietnam, Haiti, Balkans, Southwest Asia).

PTSD also frequently occurs in the presence of depression (Breslau, Davis, Peterson, & Schultz, 2000; Mollica, McIness, & Sarajliac, 1999; Shalev, Freedman, & Peri, 1998) and is associated with increased alcohol consumption (Brown & Wolfe, 1994; Zlotnick, Warshaw, & Shea, 1999). The extent to which the functional status of individuals with PTSD is influenced by comorbidity is well documented in the full PTSD population, but the current status of the subthreshold PTSD population is largely speculative and lacking evidentiary support.

PREVALENCE OF SUBTHRESHOLD PTSD

In a Canadian investigation, Stein, Walker, Hazen, and Forder (1997) observed respondents meeting subclinical criteria for PTSD reported impairment of social, occupational, and family functioning that was similar to that reported in individuals with full PTSD. Stein et al. conservatively defined subthreshold PTSD as having at least one symptom in each DSM-IV (American Psychiatric Association, 2000) symptom category. The prevalence of full PTSD in this study was 1.7 percent for men; 5.0 percent for women, and for subthreshold PTSD 2.2 percent for men and 5.7 percent for women. This pattern has been found in other "high risk" groups (Marshall et al., 2001).

PREVALENCE AND TEMPORAL DIFFERENCES

In each of the studies mentioned, comparable results held form despite the temporal differences (e.g., 20 years later in Sabin, Cardozo, Nackerud, Kaiser, & Varese, 2003; 1–4 months later in Schutzwohl & Maercker, 1999). Furthermore, in the studies of Canadian peacekeepers by Asmundson, Stein, and McCreary (2002) and Asmundson, Wright, McCreary, and Pedlar (2003), the severity of the psychopathology of respondents with subthreshold PTSD paralleled the experimental groups with full PTSD, but to a lesser degree, and was more impaired than the non-deployed or non-traumatized control group. Furthermore, two Croatian veterans' studies of 3,217 personnel showed 16.22% with current PTSD and 25% with subthreshold PTSD one year after the war (Komar & Vukusic, 1999), while the rate of current PTSD increased to 24% just one year later (Kozaric-Kovacic, 1999), suggesting that some of the subthreshold group had developed full PTSD. Weiss et al. (1992) reported a lifetime prevalence of full PTSD in 30.9% of males and 26% in females, with a lifetime prevalence of subthreshold PTSD of 22.5% and 21.2%, respectively. One point seven million respondents reported symptoms of PTSD while 49% ($n = 830,000$) of the respondents in the study still reported experiencing significant symptoms associated with PTSD in 1992. The contribution of subthreshold PTSD would add another 350,000 veterans potentially in need of treatment. Other studies with samples of veterans support this claim (Asmundson et al., 2003; Passey, 1995; Southwick et al., 1995).

The point to emphasize from the studies to date is that subthreshold PTSD, despite its varying operational definitions and temporal differences (Schutzwohl & Maercker, 1999), is about as prevalent as full PTSD and is indeed associated with substantial psychological and social impairment.

The second point and the main thrust for the present study is that, to the best of the authors' knowledge, only three previous investigations (i.e., Asmundson et al., 2003; Marshall et al., 2001; Zlotnick, Franklin, & Zimmerman, 2002), cited and addressed comorbidities, while noting subthreshold PTSD in their samples. This is key, because the level of impairment in the other studies may not be attributable to PTSD alone. High rates of comorbid disorders have been observed with PTSD (Breslau, Davis, Andreski, & Peterson, 1991; Kulka et al., 1990; Kulka et al., 1991). These studies of trauma survivors consistently show that PTSD is associated with increased psychiatric morbidity and associated impairment.

The studies of Mollica et al. (1999), Zoellner, Goodwin, and Foa (2000), and Clum, Calhoun, and Kimerling (2000) provide a foundation from which to compare the level of traumatic stress on related factors of depression, alcohol use, and physical health problems.

Operationalizing Subthreshold PTSD

Past research has shown it is the re-experiencing symptom that is important to the demarcation between full and subthreshold PTSD. In military veterans with PTSD, re-experiencing symptoms are significantly associated with current dysfunction and current disability (Beckham et al., 1997). Asmundson et al. (2003) found that symptoms of chronic pain and PTSD are significantly related to one another and, using confirmatory factor analysis (CFA), determined that it was the re-experiencing symptom that significantly separated the PTSD and subthreshold PTSD. Respondents who meet the requisite number of symptoms for cluster B plus the criteria for one other symptom cluster criteria (e.g., clusters BC, BD) will be considered to have subthreshold PTSD, while those without cluster B, one, or none of the symptom criteria (e.g., CD, B, C, D, or none) will be deemed as not having PTSD. Only respondents who meet the criteria for clusters B, C, and D will be classified as having full PTSD.

METHOD

Participants and Procedure

Participants were 1,101 male veterans (representing a response rate of approximately 72%) from regular and reserve duty forces of the Canadian military who, as part of a health status assessment conducted by Veterans' Affairs Canada in the Fall of 1999, voluntarily and anonymously completed a self-administered battery of questionnaires that included measures of PTSD symptoms, depression, alcohol use, and general health status (described in detail below). Socio-demographic and military service information was also provided. Approximately 18% of the peacekeepers met the cutoff for current PTSD on the PTSD Checklist—Military Version and another 13% met the criteria for subthreshold PTSD (Forbes, Creamer, & Biddle, 2001; Weathers, Litz, Herman, Huska, & Keane, 1993).

Measures

Participants completed socio-demographic and military service questions as well as measures of PTSD symptoms, depression, alcohol use, and health status. PTSD was assessed using established measures, while health status was evaluated using a series of questions compiled by the Veterans' Care Needs project.

PTSD CHECKLIST—MILITARY VERSION

The PTSD Checklist—Military Version (PCL-M; Weathers et al., 1993) is a self-report measure comprised of 17 items that correspond to current DSM-IV-TR (American Psychiatric Association, 2000) symptoms for PTSD. The measure yields a total score, as well as subscale scores for re-experiencing, avoidance/numbing, and hyper-arousal. The re-experiencing items of the PCL-M have been written specifically to reflect military experiences (e.g., "Repeated, disturbing memories, thoughts, or images of a stressful military experience?"). Respondents are asked to indicate the degree to which they have been bothered by each symptom over the past month, on a scale anchored from 1 (*not at all*) to 5 (*extremely*). Test—retest reliability for the PCL-M (over a 2–3 day retest interval) is .96 (Weathers et al., 1993). The PCL-M yields an adequately high overall diagnostic efficiency of .90 (Blanchard, Jones-Alexander,

Buckley, & Forneris, 1996) and has convergent validity with the Mississippi Scale for Combat-Related PTSD ($r = .93$), the PK scale of the MMPI-2 ($r = .77$), and the Impact of Event Scale ($r = .90$; Weathers et al., 1993).

THE CENTER FOR EPIDEMIOLOGICAL STUDY–DEPRESSION SCALE

The Center for Epidemiological Study–Depression Scale (CES-D; Radloff, 1977) is a 20-item measure of current (i.e., past week) depressive symptoms. Respondents rate items on a four-point scale ranging from 0 (*rarely/none of the time*) to 3 (*most/all of the time*). The measure yields a total score indicative of degree of depression. Radloff (1977) reported acceptable internal consistency (alpha > 0.84) and test–retest reliability ranging from 0.49 (12 months) to 0.67 (4 weeks). The CES-D has satisfactory convergent validity with other measures of depressive symptoms (e.g., $r > .50$ with the Hamilton Rating Scale for Depression; Devins & Orme, 1985).

Alcohol use was assessed using the Alcohol Use Disorders Identification Test (AUDIT) (Babor, de la Fuente, & Saunders, 1992). The core assessment consists of 10 multiple-choice and yes–no questions, 3 on quantity and frequency of alcohol consumption, 3 on harmful drinking, and 4 on hazardous drinking. All of the questions are scored using a 5-point Likert scale ranging from 0 (*never*) to 4 (*daily or almost daily*). The 10 items in the core questionnaire are summed to yield a total score of 0–40. A high score on the quantity and frequency items (1–3) indicates hazardous use, a high score on the second three items (4–6) implies alcohol dependence, and a high score on the remaining items (7–10) suggests harmful use.

Since the AUDIT was first published in 1989, studies have observed high internal consistency, suggesting the AUDIT measures what it purports to measure (Powell & McInness, 1994; Hays, Merz, & Nicholas, 1995). Babor et al. (1992) reported a test–retest reliability of $r = .86$ in a sample of non-hazardous drinkers, alcoholics, and cocaine abusers. Intra-scale reliability coefficients (Cronbach's alpha) were found in a cross-national sample ranging from $\alpha = .80$ in Australia to $\alpha = .98$ in Mexico (King & Bordnick, 2002). The AUDIT performs well compared to other criterion measures and, in some empirical studies, more accurately (Allen, Litten, Fertig, & Babor, 1997; Clements, 1998; Hays et al., 1995). The AUDIT correlates to the MAST (Selzer, 1971; $r = .88$) for both men and women. Correlation with the CAGE was nearly as high ($r = .78$) (Ewing, 1984).

Number of physical health problems was reported as part of a general health questionnaire.

Data Analysis

This study is a secondary data analysis. All available response data from the Regular Forces Data set pertaining to PTSD, Depression, Alcohol use, and the selected demographic variables were used in the study (e.g., *x* independent variables: PTSD [3 levels-Full, Subthreshold, No] Age; Marital Status; Years Married; Number of Deployments; Years of Service; Service Status; Rank; and Language/Ethnicity—*y* dependent variables: Depression, Alcohol problems).

RESULTS

Sample Demographics

One (Variable) by three (PTSD Status) ANOVAs were performed on all respondent continuous variables with post hoc Bonferonni tests, and 1 (Variable) by × 3 (PTSD Status); Table 1 presents a summary of the ANOVA results. Chi-square tests were conducted for all respondent categorical demographic measures. On the demographic variables pertaining to military service, there were no statistically significant differences on the following variables: Number of Deployments, Service Status, Average Number of Years Served, and Present Rank/Rank at Release from Service. These results suggest that the PTSD status groups were comparable with respect to the demographic variables associated with military service. The demographic variables pertaining to personal background showed no significant differences on Personal Income, Primary Language/Ethnicity, and Length of Marriage; however, Marital Status and Age were found to be significant.

Most of the sample was comprised of married soldiers (84.8%) and, indeed, there were significant differences for Marital Status (X^2, $p < .001$) on PTSD status. However, the literature on marital status with respect to PTSD is mixed. Studies have shown marital status as either a protective factor against vulnerability of PTSD (e.g., Sabin et al., 2003) or a source of vulnerability to PTSD (e.g., Black, 1993). Typically, marriage, as well as age, is not related to PTSD status (e.g., Birmes et al., 2001).

TABLE 1 Means, Standard Deviations, ANOVA Results on the AUDIT, CES-D, and Physical Health by PTSD Status

	PTSD Status				
	Full PTSD ($n = 207$) Mean (*SD*)	Sub-PTSD ($n = 148$) Mean (*SD*)	No PTSD ($n = 746$) Mean (*SD*)	Total ($n = 1101$) Mean (*SD*)	*F*
AUDIT	7.33 (5.40)	5.69 (3.90)	5.34 (3.42)	6.12 (4.24)	20.89
CES-D	25.16 (12.17)	14.77 (9.73)	8.53 (6.14)	12.49 (10.37)	346.29
Physical Health	3.76 (2.13)	3.05 (1.83)	2.66 (1.83)	2.92 (1.94)	27.74

Note. AUDIT = Alcohol Use Disorders Identification Test (Babor et al., 1992); CES-D = The Center for Epidemiological Study–Depression Scale (Radloff, 1977).

The overall mean age was 49.8 years old, with a standard deviation of 10.8 years, and a range from 20 to 66 years old. Age increased as PTSD symptoms decreased. For each level of traumatic stress on age, the means and standard deviations are: PTSD group ($n = 207$), $m = 44.5$, $SD = 10.4$; Subthreshold PTSD group ($n = 148$), $m = 49.0$, $SD = 10.7$; and No PTSD group ($n = 746$), $m = 50.9$, $SD = 10.5$. The one-way ANOVA for age on PTSD showed statistically significant differences, $F(2, 1098) = 33.516$, $p < .001$. Although the mean age by PTSD status was significantly different, this could be a result of the large sample size. The statistical difference was not meaningful, as less than 6% of the sample variance in PTSD status could be explained by age, (Partial $\eta^2 = .058$). However, to rule out confounding variables, an ANCOVA including Age as a covariate was run.

Overall, the results pertaining to the demographic variables suggested that the PTSD status groups were comparable.

Analysis of PTSD and Three Dependent Measures

The analysis addressed the primary research questions concerning differences in PTSD status on three dependent measures. The dependent variables were assessed in four parts. First, each is evaluated with a one-way-ANOVA to determine if there are overall main effects for PTSD status on the dependent variable. Second, the means and standard deviations are reported for PTSD status on the dependent measure. Third, when significant main effects were found, post hoc analyses using the Bonferonni method to control for Type I error were done to make pairwise comparisons of PTSD status (using a Bonferroni-corrected alpha, $p = .01667$). Finally, a one-way ANCOVA was done using age as a covariate to determine if age could explain any of the differences on the outcome measures.

The ANOVA results indicate alcohol problems, $F(2, 1098) = 20.893$, $p < .001$, depressive symptoms, $F(2, 1098) = 346.285$, $p < .001$, and number of physical health problems, $F(2, 1098) = 27.736$, $p < .001$, differentiated the three PTSD status groups. To demonstrate a meaningful difference between the population means the effect size, partial omega squared (ω^2), was calculated. The differences on CES-D (partial $\omega^2 = .39$) were moderate, while on the AUDIT (partial $\omega^2 = .03$) and number of physical health problems (partial $\omega^2 = .05$), differences were small.

Because a main effect was found on Number of Alcohol Use disorders, Depressive Symptoms, and Number of Physical Health Problems, a series of follow-up pairwise comparisons were computed to examine contrasts between the three groups (Full, Subthreshold, and No PTSD). Full PTSD was significantly different from No PTSD on Alcohol, Use Depression, and Number of Physical Health Problems ($p < .001$). Subthreshold PTSD was significantly different from Full PTSD ($p < .001$) on all three dependent measures. Finally, Subthreshold PTSD was significantly different from the

No PTSD group ($p < .001$) on Depression and Number of Physical Health Problems, but not statistically significantly different ($p = .950$) on Alcohol Use disorders.

Finally, a one-way analysis of covariance (ANCOVA) was conducted to determine if Age could explain differences on the AUDIT, CESD, and on Number of Physical Health Problems. The ANCOVA indicated that the relationship between the covariate and two of the dependent variables (AUDIT) did not differ significantly as a function of PTSD status: AUDIT, $F(1, 1097, .05) = .002$, $p = .967$; Number of Physical Health Problems, $F(1, 1097, .05) < .001$, $p = .950$. Thus, Age was not determined to be an influential factor on Alcohol Use. The ANCOVA indicated that the relationship between the covariate and the dependent variable (CESD) remained significant, $F(1, 1097, .05) = .6.866$, $p = .009$, partial $\eta^2 = .006$). The low effect size shows that the statistical difference is not a meaningful one.

DISCUSSION

The findings of this study suggest that veterans with Full and Subthreshold forms of PTSD have higher levels of depression and health problems than veterans with no PTSD. When looking at Subthreshold PTSD more closely, veterans appear to have higher levels of psychiatric and physical morbidity compared to their normal (No PTSD) counterparts, but not to the extent of those veterans diagnosed with Full posttraumatic stress disorder. These findings warrant further discussion.

PTSD symptoms and poor health in military veterans has been discussed in the literature for the past several years (Asmundson et al., 2002; Beckham et al., 1998; Hotopf, 2003; Kimerling et al., 2000; Shigemura & Nomura, 2002; Wagner et al., 2000). Research involving links between alcohol abuse (Brown and Wolfe, 1994; Mehlum, 1998; Wedding, 1987; Zlotnick et al., 1999) and depression (Boisvert, McCreary, Wright, & Asmundsen, 2003; Breslau et al., 2000; Mollica et al., 1999; Shalev et al., 1998). Have been examined in terms of relationship to PTSD symptoms, in the biological and behavioral treatment areas. The primary purpose of this investigation was to extend these findings by comparing groups of peacekeepers with Full, Subthreshold, and No PTSD on measures of Alcohol Use Disorders, Depression and Physical Health Problems. The main findings of this study will now be discussed, with a secondary emphasis on the relationship of Subthreshold PTSD to groups with Full PTSD or No PTSD.

The main findings of this study were as follows:

- Peacekeepers with Full PTSD were statistically significantly different from those with Subthreshold PTSD and No PTSD in level of impairment on the measure of Alcohol Use Disorders.

- Peacekeepers with Full PTSD were statistically significantly different from those with Subthreshold PTSD and No PTSD in level of impairment on the measure for Depressive symptoms.
- Peacekeepers with Subthreshold PTSD had generally higher mean levels of impairment than those with No PTSD on all three dependent measures.
- Peacekeepers with current Subthreshold PTSD did not significantly differ from those with No PTSD on the AUDIT in degree of Alcohol Use Disorders, but were significantly different than those with Full PTSD.
- Peacekeepers with Subthreshold PTSD, compared to those with Full PTSD, were significantly different from the No PTSD group on the CESD, suggesting that people with Subthreshold PTSD are more depressed compared to those with No PTSD, but were also statistically significantly different from the Full PTSD group, suggesting they are not as comparable to peacekeepers with Full PTSD as hypothesized.
- PTSD influences health status. Peacekeepers in the Full PTSD group had more physical health problems than those in the No PTSD group and, as one would expect, the older veterans with PTSD had higher means than their younger counterparts.
- Deployed and Non-deployed peacekeepers were both represented in the Full and Subthreshold PTSD groups, suggesting that PTSD could occur as a result of both domestic and foreign service.

Previous research by King and Bordnick (2002) recognized that research on PTSD should put the disorder into the context of the veteran's life. The current study broadened the understanding of PTSD of Canadian veterans of U.N. peacekeeping missions by comparing groups of veterans with varying PTSD statuses on alcohol use disorders, depressive symptoms, and physical health problems. The results will now be discussed for the three dependent measures.

Alcohol Use Disorders

Scores on measures of current PTSD symptoms (PCL-M) and Alcohol Use Disorders (AUDIT) were compared across three groups of veterans with varying PTSD statuses. It was hypothesized that peacekeepers in the Full or Subthreshold PTSD groups would have more severe Alcohol Use scores. The results were as expected, with the Full PTSD group having the highest levels of Alcohol Use and the Subthreshold PTSD group having the second highest mean.

The results for Alcohol Use are consistent with other international veteran studies (Bleich, Siegei, Garb, & Lerer, 1986; Lerer, 1987; Spivak, Segal, Laufer, Mester, & Weitzman, 2000), showing lower alcohol use disorder mean scores than in the United States. This finding may be explained by the lack of Vietnam-era veterans in the VAC system. The present data supports the suggestion that the link between military induced-PTSD and alcohol abuse may reflect a cultural norm and that the particularly high association between combat-related PTSD may be unique to the Vietnam experience (Lerer et al., 1987; Spivak et al., 2000).

Past research by McFall, Makcay, and Donovan (1992) showed that PTSD influences alcohol use patterns in veterans. Likewise, this study found significant differences between PTSD status when comparing Alcohol Use disorders. It was expected that veterans with full PTSD and subthreshold PTSD would have clinical levels of Alcohol Use disorders. This hypothesis was based on the idea that the natural course of alcohol abuse parallels the course of PTSD (Bremner, Southwick, Darnell, & Charney, 1996) and, like combat veterans, Canadian peacekeepers have increased alcohol consumption as PTSD status increased. The hypothesis was not supported because Alcohol Use was not significantly different between the Subthreshold and No PTSD groups. However, expected trends were clearly observable, as drinking behavior did increase with severity of PTSD status. Previous research on Canadian peacekeepers with PTSD showed higher rates of alcohol abuse among the peacekeepers with PTSD (Passey, 1995).

Past research findings by Skinner and Allen (1982) show that the degree of alcohol dependence on PTSD is directly related to psychopathology and to physical symptoms of the nervous, cardiovascular, and digestive systems of veterans. In the following sections, the current findings on depression and physical health problems showed significant differences with the full PTSD groups having the greatest impairment, supporting the findings of Skinner and Allen.

Depression

Scores on measures of current PTSD symptoms (PCL-M) and depressive symptoms (CESD) were compared. It was hypothesized that peacekeepers with Full or Subthreshold PTSD would have more severe Depression scores. The results were nearly as expected, with the Full PTSD group having clinical levels of depressive symptoms and the Subthreshold PTSD group approaching clinical levels of depressive symptoms.

These results are consistent with other research findings on depression and veterans. In similar comparison studies, severity of trauma was the best predictor of the severity in the outcome measures for depression (Bleich, Koslowsky, & Lerer, 1997; Clum et al., 2000). Bleich et al.'s (1997) study found that major depressive disorder was the most common concomitant diagnosis, with a lifetime prevalence of 95% and current prevalence of 50%. In a study by Stein and Kennedy (2001), 42.9% of the cases with PTSD had major depressive disorder. This study's findings support observations by McQuaid, Pedrelli, McCahill, and Stein (2001) in which 23% of the respondents who met criteria for full or subthreshold PTSD met the criteria for major depressive disorder. Finally, Asmundson et al. (2002) found that PTSD symptoms contributed to depression in Canadian peacekeepers. Asmundson et al. also found that PTSD influenced health status through depression. In follow-up research, Asmundson et al. (2003) found that PTSD significantly influences chronic pain. This finding led to the current investigation's interest in PTSD with respect to the number of physical health problems reported by Canadian peacekeepers.

Physical Health

Studies by Mollica et al. (1999), Zoellner et al. (2000), and Clum et al. (2000) provided the foundation from which to compare and evaluate influences of PTSD symptoms and related physical factors on health status. There have, to the best of our knowledge, been only two investigations of this sort on military personnel deployed to peacekeeping missions and war zones. The first, by Schnurr and Spiro (1999), indicated that PTSD had a direct influence on physical health status. The second, by Asmundson et al. (2002), found that PTSD symptoms directly influenced health status and indirectly influenced depression. They also found that PTSD influenced alcohol use. This investigation extended these findings.

When comparing PTSD status on a number of health problems, depressive symptoms, and alcohol use disorders, the more severe the PTSD the higher the mean score on the outcome measure. Full PTSD had the highest mean scores on each, followed by Subthreshold PTSD, and No PTSD respectively. Since the Subthreshold PTSD group was found to be significantly different in most cases from the No PTSD group on each dependent measure, subthreshold PTSD is discussed further.

Subthreshold PTSD

One purpose of this study was to look more closely at subthreshold PTSD. The results had several important implications. First, the findings of this study support the findings of research by Zlotnick et al. (2002), as the present research demonstrates that subthreshold PTSD is associated with psychological morbidity and is an indicator of impairment in peacekeepers to a lesser degree than full PTSD. Second, levels of impairment on Depression and Health Problems approached the levels for those peacekeepers with full PTSD, as was the case in Boisvert et al. (2003), highlighting the importance of subthreshold PTSD as a meaningful indicator of psychiatric morbidity. Finally, although the overall findings lend support to the validity of the current diagnostic thresholds for full PTSD, they also indicate that subthreshold PTSD is a meaningful diagnosis, as subthreshold PTSD significantly impacts the affect and mental health of the peacekeeping veteran. For example, a substantial proportion (30.3%) of veterans with Subthreshold PTSD reported clinical levels of depression. This latter finding supports the notion that clinical problems are indeed associated with subthreshold PTSD and suggests that clinical attention to and intervention for subthreshold PTSD would be beneficial for veterans. Likewise, the fact that subthreshold symptoms have persisted beyond the veterans' service, appear to occur with near clinical levels of depression, demonstrate poorer health than those without PTSD and are at levels comparable to veterans with full PTSD warrants further attention. Studies involving a temporal model of PTSD are also warranted.

The current study was both similar to and different from previous studies, such as the definition of subthreshold PTSD and the nature of the respondents in the sample. Unlike the Zlotnick et al. (2002) sample, Subthreshold PTSD in this study was significantly different from No PTSD on some measures of psychiatric impairment, namely the CESD and health. Similar to this study, Asmundson et al. (2003) and Zlotnick et al. (2002) found that patients with subthreshold PTSD had the re-experiencing criterion plus symptoms from one other diagnostic cluster. Since 12.1% of the sample met criteria for two of three symptom clusters and appeared impaired, the issue of whether or not the current diagnostic thresholds for PTSD are too stringent persists. While veterans with Full PTSD were more impaired (as expected), the results of veterans with Subthreshold PTSD on depression suggests they should receive clinical attention for symptoms of both depression and PTSD.

In contrast to Zlotnick et al. (2002), this study used military veterans rather than civilian psychiatric patients. Since this study used veterans of potentially dangerous military missions rather than civilian psychiatric patients, it is possible that the reason the Subthreshold and No PTSD groups were not always significantly different was an overall baseline of distress existed, as indicated by the CESD. The present study did substantiate this in that it used a sample of treatment-seeking veterans that were already VAC pensioners. Therefore, differences between the Subthreshold PTSD and the No PTSD groups on the AUDIT, for example, might be less apparent.

Arguments against the importance of subthreshold PTSD could look to the fact that the present study observed that full PTSD was significantly different compared to both Subthreshold PTSD and No PTSD on the indices of psychiatric morbidity. This finding suggests that full PTSD impacts the intensity of symptoms of other diagnoses more so than subthreshold PTSD, yet it does not mean that subthreshold PTSD does not have a marked effect on those veterans with comorbidity. What it does suggest is an indicator that the boundary between PTSD and other psychiatric diagnoses is valid.

Limitations

GENERALIZABILITY

There are several limitations to this study. The results of this study may not generalize to other traumatized populations, such as the general population, civilian psychiatric patients, or victims of other types of trauma, such as motor vehicle accidents. This study was also limited to male peacekeepers and may not generalize to female soldiers. This sample may not be representative of PTSD prevalence rates in the Canadian forces in general because the sample is comprised of VAC treatment-seeking pensioners. Another limitation is intrinsic to the screening instrument used to capture the construct of PTSD: the question in this investigation's survey version of the PCL-M asking veterans if they experienced a life-threatening event is missing. As a result, it can only be said that peacekeepers meeting subthreshold or full diagnostic levels of PTSD have "probable PTSD" (Asmundson et al., 2003).

PROCEDURAL CONSIDERATIONS

There were four methodological limitations in the present study. The use of secondary data and retrospective measures may have obscured some of the findings because there is no baseline of how these veterans looked prior to engaging in their peacekeeping missions (i.e., did the exposure to trauma precede peacekeeping?). The lack of data specifying traumatic events and age of onset limits the interpretation of the findings. Without this data, the type and severity of the veterans' traumatic experiences remains uncertain, impacting the interpretation of the findings on issues such as the impact of deploying. However, the fact that the symptoms have persisted until the time of the study is worth noting due to the fact that over 30% of the sample has probable PTSD or subthreshold PTSD. Finally, the use of secondary data to study the concept of subthreshold PTSD does not address the predictive validity of the concept or provide empirical cause to treat subthreshold PTSD. These findings suggest that subthreshold PTSD is an indicator that there are many more impaired veterans due to trauma than perhaps previously thought.

Future Research

Several things must be studied in the future. Longitudinal studies are required to examine whether the presence of subthreshold PTSD prolongs the duration of health-related problems and increases the risk of the onset of full PTSD and other psychiatric disorders. Subthreshold PTSD also appears to have a persistent quality, thus distinguishing it from normal responses to trauma. A study of the temporal aspect of subthreshold PTSD and impairment also needs study. Finally, demographic information was studied to determine how personal characteristics influences the differences within the grouping variable on measures of psychiatric morbidity. The next logical step would be to look at what demographic factors place one at risk for full or subthreshold PTSD.

CONCLUSION

The findings of this study are consistent with previous empirical investigations of subthreshold PTSD. They highlight the importance of expanding research beyond the taxometric criteria for PTSD. The study, while showing that the current thresholds for PTSD do indicate greater severity of comorbid psychiatric problems, fuels the on-going debate associated with nosological approaches to sequelae of posttraumatic stress disorder. The present investigation calls attention to an important military and public health implication that greater numbers of veterans and civilians may experience disability than previously thought because of expanding PTSD rates beyond the threshold of full PTSD. Longitudinal studies are needed which monitor soldiers from entrance into the military through subsequent military experience until retirement. Further, clinical trials of subthreshold PTSD and comorbidity need examination in the near future to further evaluate the relative importance of subthreshold disorders.

ACKNOWLEDGEMENT

Thank you to Veterans Affairs Canada, Charlottetown, PEI for making available the 1999 Regular Forces Dataset for research.

REFERENCES

Allen, J. P., Litten, R. Z., Fertig, J. B., and Babor, T. F. (1997). A review of research on Alcohol Use Disorders Identification Test (AUDIT). *Alcoholism: Clinical and Experimental Research, 21*(4), 613–619.

American Psychiatric Association. (1980). *Diagnostic and statistical manual of mental disorders, 3rd Ed.* Washington, D.C.: Author.

American Psychiatric Association. (2000). *Diagnostic and statistical manual of mental disorders, 4th Ed.* Washington, D.C.: Author.

Asmundson, G. J. G., Stein, M. B., and McCreary, D. (2002). PTSD symptoms influence health status of deployed peacekeepers and non-deployed personnel. *Journal of Nervous and Mental Disease, 190*(12), 807–815.

Asmundson, G. J. G., Wright, K., McCreary, D., and Pedlar, D. (2003). Posttraumatic stress disorder symptoms in United Nations peacekeepers: An examination of factor structure and the influence of chronic pain. *Cognitive Behaviour Therapy, 32*(1), 26–37.

Babor, T. F., de la Fuente, J. R., and Saunders, J. (1992). *AUDIT, The Alcohol Use Disorders Identification Test: Guidelines for use in primary health care.* (PSA/92.4). Geneva: World Health Organization.

Beckham, J. C., Crawford, A. L., Feldman, M. E., Kirby, A. C., Hertzberg, M. A., Davidson, J. R., et al. (1997). Chronic posttraumatic stress disorder and chronic pain in Vietnam veterans. *Journal of Psychosomatic Research, 43*(4), 379–389.

Beckham, J. C., Moore, S. D., Feldman, M. E., Herzberg, M. A., Kirby, A. C., and Fairbank, J. A. (1998). Health status, somatization and posttraumatic stress disorder severity in Vietnam combat veterans with posttraumatic stress disorder. *The American Journal of Psychiatry, 155*, 1565–1569.

Birmes, P., Carreras, D., Ducassé, J., Charlet, J., Warner, B. A., Lauque, D., et al. (2001). Peritraumatic dissociation, acute stress, and early posttraumatic stress disorder in victims of general crime. *Canadian Journal of Psychiatry, 46*(7), 649–651.

Black, W. G. (1993). Military-induced family separation. *Social Work, 38*, 273–280.

Blanchard, E. B., Jones-Alexander, J., Buckley, T. C., and Forneris, C. A. (1996). Psychometric properties of the PTSD Checklist (PCL). *Behavior Research and Therapy, 34*, 669–673.

Bleich, A., Koslowsky, A. D., and Lerer, B. (1997). Post-traumatic stress disorder and depression: An analysis of comorbidity. *British Journal of Psychiatry, 170*, 479–482.

Bleich, A., Siegei, B., Garb, R., and Lerer, B. (1986). Post-traumatic stress disorder following combat exposure. *British Journal of Psychiatry, 149*, 365–369

Boisvert, J. A., McCreary, D., Wright, K., and Asmundson, G. J. G. (2003). Factor validity of the Center for Epidemiologic Studies Depression (CES-D) Scale in military peacekeepers. *Depression and Anxiety, 17*, 19–25.

Bremner, D. J., Southwick, S., Darnell, A., and Charney, D. S. (1996). Chronic PTSD in Vietnam combat veterans: course of illness and substance abuse. *American Journal of Psychiatry, 153*(3), 369–375.

Breslau, N., Davis, G. C., Andreski, P., and Peterson, E. L. (1991). Traumatic events and posttraumatic stress disorder in an urban population of young adults. *Archives in General Psychiatry, 48*, 216–222.

Breslau, N., Davis, G. C., Peterson, E. L., and Schultz, L. R. (2000). A second look at comorbidity in victims of trauma: The posttraumatic stress disorder - major depression connection. *Biological Psychiatry, 48*, 902–909.

Brown, P. J. and Wolfe, J. (1994). Substance abuse and post-traumatic stress disorder comorbidity. *Drug and Alcohol Dependency, 35*, 51–59.

Clements, R. (1998). A critical evaluation of several alcohol screening instruments using the CIDI-SAM as a criterion measure. *Alcoholism: Clinical and Experimental Research, 22*(5), 985–993.

Clum, G. A., Calhoun, K. S., and Kimerling, R. (2000). Associations among symptoms of depression and posttraumatic stress disorder and self-reported health in sexually assaulted women. *Journal of Nervous and Mental Disease, 188*, 671–678.

Devins, G. M. and Orme, C. M. (1985). Center for epidemiologic studies depression scale. In D. J. Keyser and R. C. Sweetland (Eds.), *Test critiques:* Vol. 2. Kansas City, MO: Test Corporation of America.

Ewing, J. A. (1984). Detecting alcoholism: The CAGE questionnaire. *Journal of the American Medical Association, 252*, 1905–1907.

Forbes, D., Creamer, M., and Biddle, D. (2001). The validity of the PTSD checklist as a measure of symptomatic change in combat-related PTSD. *Behaviour Research and Therapy, 39*, 977–986.

Hathaway, S. R. and McKinley, J. C. (1989). *MMPI-2 (Minnesota Multiphasic Personality Inventory-2)*. University of Minnesota Press.

Hays, R. D., Merz, J. F., and Nicholas, R. (1995). Response burden, reliability, and validity of the CAGE, Short MAST, and AUDIT alcohol screening measures. *Behavioral Research Methods, Instruments and Computers, 27*, 277–280.

Hotopf, M., David, A. S., Hull, L., Ismail, K., Palmer, I., Unwin, C., et al. (2003). The health effects of peace-keeping in UK Armed Forces: Bosnia 1992–1996. Predictors of Psychological Symptoms. *Psychological Medicine, 33*, 155–162.

Kimerling, R., Clum, G. A., and Wolfe, J. (2000). Relationships among trauma exposure, chronic posttraumatic stress disorder symptoms, and self-reported health in women: Replication and extension. *Journal of Traumatic Stress, 13*, 115–128.

King, M. E. and Bordnick, P. S. (2002). Alcohol use disorders: A social worker's guide to clinical assessment. *Journal of Social Work Practice in the Addictions, 2*(1), 3–31.

Komar, Z. and Vukusic, H. (1999). Posttraumatic stress disorder in Croatia war veterans: Prevalence and psycho-social characteristics. In D. Dekaris and A. Sabioncello (Eds.), *New insight in posttraumatic stress disorder (PTSD)* (pp. 42–44). Zagreb, Croatia: Croatian Academy of Science and Arts.

Kozaric-Kovacic, D. (1999). PTSD and comorbidity. In D. Dekaris and A. Sabioncello (Eds.), *New insight in posttraumatic stress disorder (PTSD)*. Zagreb, Croatia: Croatian Academy of Science and Arts.

Kulka, R. A., Schlenger, W. E., Fairbank, J. A., Hough, R. L., Jordan, B. K., Marmar, C. R., et al. (1990). *Trauma and the Vietnam war generation*. New York: Brunner/Mazel.

Kulka, R. A., Schlenger, W. E., Fairbank, J. A., Hough, B. K., Marmar, C. R., and Weiss, D. S. (1991). Assessment of PTSD in the community: Prospects and pitfalls from recent studies of Vietnam veterans. *Journal of Consulting and Clinical Psychology, 3*, 547–560.

Lerer, B., Bleich, A., Kotler, M., Garb, R., Hertzberg, M. A., and Levin, B. (1987). Post-traumatic stress disorder in Israeli combat veterans. *Archives in General Psychiatry, 44*, 976–981.

Marshall, R. D., Olfson, M., Hellman, F., Blanco, C., Guardino, M., and Struening, E. L. (2001). Comorbidity, impairment and suicidality in subthreshold PTSD. *American Journal of Psychiatry, 158*, 1467–1473.

Marshall, R. P., Jorm, A. F., and Grayson, D. A. (1998). Posttraumatic stress disorder and other predictors of health care consumption by Vietnam veterans. *Psychiatric Services, 49*, 1609–1611.

McFall, M., Makcay, P., and Donovan, D. (1992). Combat-related post-traumatic stress disorder and severity of substance abuse in Vietnam veterans. *Journal of Studies of Alcohol, 53*, 357–363.

McQuaid, J. R., Pedrelli, P., McCahill, M. E., and Stein, M. B. (2001). Reported trauma, post-traumatic stress disorder and major depression among primary care patients. *Psychological Medicine, 31*, 1249–1257.

Mehlum, L. (1998). *Alcohol and stress in Norwegian UN peace-keepers*. Paper presented at the International conference on the psycho-social consequences of war, Dubrovnik, Croatia.

Mollica, R. F., McIness, K., and Sarajliac, N. (1999). Disability associated with psychiatric comorbidity and health status in Bosnian refugees living in Croatia. *Journal of the American Medical Association, 282,* 433–439.

Passey, G. (1995). *Psychological consequences of Canadian U.N. peacekeeping duties in Croatia and Bosnia 1992–93.* Paris, France: 4th European Conference on Traumatic Stress.

Powell, J. E. and McInness, K. (1994). Alcohol use among older hospital patients: Findings from an Australian study. *Drug and Alcohol Review, 13,* 5–12.

Radloff, L. (1977). The CES-D Scale: A self-report depression scale for research in the general population. *Applied Psychological Measures, 1,* 385–401.

Resnick, H. S., Acierno, R., and Kilpatrick, D. G. (1997). Health impact of internal personal violence 2: Medical and mental health outcomes. *Behavioral Medicine, 23,* 65–78.

Sabin, M., Cardozo, B. L., Nackerud, L., Kaiser, R., and Varese, L. (2003). *Guatemalan refugees twenty years later: Factors associated with poor mental health outcomes.* Unpublished manuscript accepted by JAMA, Athens, GA.

Schlenger, W. E., Fairbank, J. A., Jordan, B. K., and Caddell. (1999). Combat-related posttraumatic stress disorder: Prevalence, risk factors and comorbidity. In P. A. Saigh and J. D. Bremner (Eds.), *Posttraumatic stress disorder: A comprehensive text.* Boston: Allyn and Bacon.

Schnurr, P. P. and Jankowski, M. K. (1999). Physical health and post-traumatic stress disorder: Review and synthesis. *Seminars in Clinical Neuropsychiatry, 4,* 295–304.

Schnurr, P. P. and Spiro, A., III. (1999). Combat exposure, PTSD symptoms, and health behaviors as predictors of self-reported physical health status in older veterans. *Journal of Nervous and Mental Disease, 187,* 353–359.

Schutzwohl, M. and Maercker, A. (1999). Effects of varying diagnostic criteria for posttraumatic stress disorder are endorsing the concept of partial PTSD. *Journal of Traumatic Stress, 12*(1).

Selzer, M. L. (1971). The Michigan Alcoholism Screening Test: The quest for a new diagnostic instrument. *American Journal of Psychiatry, 127,* 1653–1656.

Shalev, A. Y., Freedman, S., and Peri, T. (1998). Prospective study of posttraumatic stress disorder and depression following trauma. *American Journal of Psychiatry, 155,* 630–637.

Shigemura, J. and Nomura, S. (2002). Mental health issues of peacekeeping workers. *Psychiatry and Clinical Neurosciences, 56,* 483–491.

Skinner, H. and Allen, B. (1982). Alcohol dependence syndrome: measurement and validation. *Journal of Abnormal Psychology, 91*(3), 199–209.

Southwick, S. M., Morgan, C. A., Darnell, A., Bremner, D. J., Nicolau, A. L., Nagy, L. M., et al. (1993). Trauma-related Symptoms in veterans of Operation Desert Storm: A 2-year Follow up. *American Journal of Psychiatry, 152*(8), 1150–1158.

Spivak, B., Segal, M., Laufer, N., Mester, R., and Weitzman, A. (2000). Lifetime psychiatric morbidity rate in Israel non-help-seeking patients with combat-related post-traumatic stress disorder. *Journal of Affective Disorders, 57,* 185–188.

Stein, M. B. and Kennedy, C. (2001). Major depressive and post-traumatic stress disorder comorbidity in female victims of intimate partner violence. *Journal of Affective Disorders, 66,* 133–138.

Stein, M. B., Walker, J. R., Hazen, A. L., and Forder, D. R. (1997). Full and partial posttraumatic stress disorder: Findings from a community survey. *American Journal of Psychiatry, 154*(8), 1114–1119.

Wagner, A. W., Wolfe, J., Rotnitsky, A., et al. (2000). An investigation of the impact of posttraumatic stress disorder on physical health. *Journal of Traumatic Stress, 13*, 41–55.

Weathers, F. W., Litz, B., Herman, D. S., Huska, J. A., and Keane, T. M. (1993). *The PTSD Checklist: Reliability, validity, and diagnostic utility*. San Antonio, TX: Paper presented at the Annual Meeting of the International Society for Traumatic Stress Studies.

Wedding, D. (1987). Substance abuse in the Vietnam veteran. *AAOHN Journal, 35*, 74–76.

Weiss, D. S., Marmar, C. R., Schlenger, W. E., Fairbank, J. A., Jordan, B. K., Hough, R. L., et al. (1992). The prevalence of lifetime and partial post-traumatic stress disorder in Vietnam theater veterans. *Journal of Traumatic Stress, 5*(3), 365–376.

Zatzick, D., Marmar, C. R., and Weiss, D. S. (1997). Posttraumatic stress disorder and functioning and quality of life outcomes in a nationally representative sample of male Vietnam veterans. *American Journal of Psychiatry, 154*, 1690–1694.

Zlotnick, C., Franklin, C. L., and Zimmerman, M. (2002). Does "subthreshold" posttraumatic stress disorder have any clinical relevance? *Comprehensive Psychiatry, 43*(6), 413–419.

Zlotnick, C., Warshaw, M., and Shea, M. T. (1999). Chronicity in posttraumatic stress disorder (PTSD) and predictors of course of comorbid PTSD in patients with anxiety disorders. *Journal of Traumatic Stress, 12*, 89–100.

Zoellner, L. A., Goodwin, M. L., and Foa, E. B. (2000). PTSD severity and health perceptions in female victims of sexual assault. *Journal of Traumatic Stress, 13*, 635–649.

Index

Printed and bound by CPI Group (UK) Ltd, Croydon, CR0 4YY

01/11/2024

01782610-0009